DK

Medical Association

FAMILY DOCTOR GUIDE *to*

SKIN AND SUNLIGHT

The British Medical Association

FAMILY DOCTOR GUIDE *to*

SKIN AND SUNLIGHT

PROFESSOR JOHN HAWK AND DR. JANE MCGREGOR

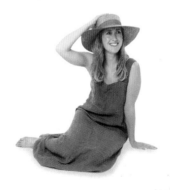

MEDICAL EDITOR
DR. TONY SMITH

A DORLING KINDERSLEY BOOK

IMPORTANT

This book is not designed as a substitute for personal medical advice but as a supplement to that advice for the patient who wishes to understand more about his/her condition.

Before taking any form of treatment YOU SHOULD ALWAYS CONSULT YOUR MEDICAL PRACTITIONER.

In particular (without limit) you should note that advances in medical science occur rapidly, and some of the information contained in this book about drugs and treatment may very soon be out of date.

PLEASE NOTE

The authors regret that they cannot enter into any correspondence with readers.

DORLING KINDERSLEY
LONDON, NEW YORK, AUCKLAND, DELHI,
JOHANNESBURG, MUNICH, PARIS AND SYDNEY

DK www.dk.com

Senior Editors Nicki Lampon, Mary Lindsay
Senior Designers Jan English, Sarah Hall
Production Controller Elizabeth Cherry

Managing Editor Martyn Page
Managing Art Editor Bryn Walls

Produced for Dorling Kindersley Limited by
Design Revolution, Queens Park Villa,
30 West Drive, Brighton, East Sussex BN2 2GE
Editorial Director Ian Whitelaw
Art Director Becky Willis
Editor Julie Whitaker
Designers Andrew Easton, Mark Batley

Published in Great Britain in 2000 by
Dorling Kindersley Limited,
9 Henrietta Street, London WC2E 8PS

2 4 6 8 10 9 7 5 3 1

A CIP catalogue record for this book is available from the British Library

ISBN: 07513 08145

Reproduced by Colourscan, Singapore
Printed in Hong Kong by Wing King Tong

Contents

Introduction

Warnings by doctors that sunlight and sunbathing can be dangerous are comparatively new. Only in the past 20 or so years have health educators tried to discourage people from exposing their bodies to too much sunlight; until then, a suntan was seen by many people as a sign of good health.

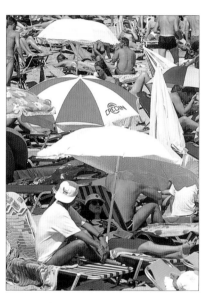

ENJOYING THE SUNSHINE
Many people have ignored the warnings about sunbathing, believing that a tan makes them feel and look healthier.

Even now, however, some people prefer to ignore these warnings because they enjoy sunbathing and believe that a tan makes them feel and look better. They therefore try to make the most of fine days by getting out in the sun as much as possible. However, the truth is that too much exposure to the sun is not good for our skins. In fact, a suntan is visible evidence of permanent damage that may ultimately lead to skin ageing and cancer.

The aim of this book is to explain how the action of sun-light on your skin leads to these changes, causing both short- and long-term damage, and to give practical advice on how to prevent such injury. Following this advice does not mean denying yourself the delights of sunshine altogether, but rather it will help you to enjoy them more safely.

Our taste for a suntan is relatively new: as recently as 100 years ago most people wanted a pale skin. Working people who spent their days out of doors became tanned and weather-beaten; the rich and fashionable preferred to avoid sunlight, wearing large hats and carrying sunshades, and saw pale complexions as a social and fashion asset. Northern Europeans certainly visited the south of France and Italy to escape the worst of the winter, but they still avoided the Mediterranean sun during the summer months.

Attitudes began to change in the 1930s as people started to enjoy outdoor recreations more – walking, camping and cycling, for example – and a suntan gradually became desirable for many people of both sexes. After World War II, cheap package holidays allowed more and more people to spend a couple of weeks soaking up the sun on Mediterranean shores, and beaches became even more popular holiday destinations in the USA, Australasia and South Africa.

It was around this time in Australia, however, that alarms were eventually sounded, attention being drawn to the high rate of skin cancers in white-skinned people living in Queensland, although European researchers had mentioned the possibility of such problems since the start of the twentieth century. Public health campaigns were started to encourage people to avoid too much exposure to strong sunlight, to use sunscreens and to learn to recognise skin cancers at an early stage. Evidence from around the world also showed that such cancers, and melanoma in particular, were rapidly becoming more common, doubling in frequency every 12 years or so; yet many people still chose to ignore these warnings. Further, in the last two decades there have also been ever-increasing suggestions that depletion of the ozone layer by atmospheric pollution is leading steadily to sunlight becoming even more dangerous; fortunately, scientists are not yet convinced that this is true, but it will become so if we do not take more care from now on.

Repeated exposure to sunlight causes photoageing of the skin – dryness, brown and red blotchiness, sagging and wrinkling – especially in people with fair skin. In addition, it may lead to skin cancers, which are now some of the most common cancers worldwide. There are some 40,000 new cases each year in the UK, including about 4,000 cases of malignant melanoma, which is responsible for about 75 per cent of the 2,000 annual deaths from skin cancer. It is an especially significant cause of death in those aged 26–35 who are otherwise relatively healthy, yet doctors estimate that around 90 per cent of all skin cancers are potentially preventable by taking care in the sun.

Later chapters in this book describe how you can recognise skin cancer in its early stages, when treatment is extremely likely to be successful. Advice is also given about the prevention of such cancers, as well as the prevention of sunburn and photoageing, and about the value of sunscreens. It is especially important to protect your children against the sun (see p.59), because they are unaware of its dangers, and exposure in early life is thought likely to play a relatively more important part in the later development of skin cancer.

Sunlight does, however, lift the spirits hugely, especially after a long dark winter. However, the rays responsible for this are probably not the damaging ultraviolet ones, but rather those usually safe ones that bring warmth and light. The advice in this book is therefore intended to help you to enjoy the great psychological and other benefits of sunshine without suffering its hidden harmful effects.

KEY POINTS

- A suntan is visible evidence of damage to the skin.
- The long-term effects of exposure to the sun can include skin ageing and cancer.
- There are some 40,000 new cases of skin cancer in the UK every year.

Solar radiation

Sunlight is so-called electromagnetic radiation – energy of many different wavelengths emitted by the sun; it travels through space at the enormous speed of 186,000 miles per second. Such energy provides us with the heat and light we need, as well as delivering damaging ultraviolet (UV) rays.

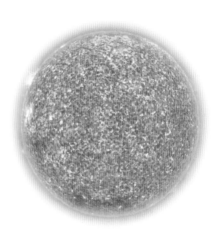

The way in which the sun's radiation affects us depends on its wavelength, which determines how it is absorbed by the molecules in our different tissues. These tissues include those in the eye responsible for vision and those in the skin, all of which are susceptible to UV injury.

SOLAR RADIATION
Electromagnetic radiation emitted by the sun provides us with the light and heat that support life on Earth but also includes damaging ultraviolet radiation.

WHAT IS SUNLIGHT?

In addition to UV, visible and infrared radiation (heat), sunlight is composed of a host of other solar rays, such as cosmic rays, gamma rays, X-rays and radiofrequency radiation, but these are present in too small quantities at the surface of the Earth, or are of too low energy, to affect our skin. When these rays penetrate the Earth's atmosphere, they are modified in various ways. For example, visible light is scattered by atmospheric oxygen and nitrogen molecules in such a way that it makes the sky look blue; in addition, some of the overall radiation energy is absorbed and some reflected back into space by these molecules, as well as by atmospheric water vapour, dust particles and other constituents. The result is that only about two-thirds of the solar energy arriving at the surface of the atmosphere penetrates to ground level, and this is made up of about five per cent UV, 40 per cent visible and 55 per cent infrared radiation.

WHY SUNLIGHT IS IMPORTANT

The energy from sunlight has been essential for the evolution of life on Earth. It has provided visible light for photosynthesis, the process by which plants use such energy to grow and eventually provide food for other creatures via the food chain. In addition, infrared rays have given us the warmth we need to live, while visible light is the part of the spectrum that our eyes need to see and that drives our biological, so-called circadian,

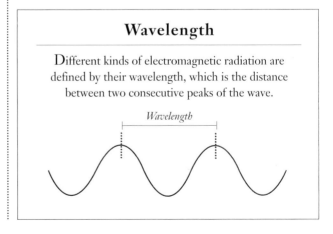

Wavelength

Different kinds of electromagnetic radiation are defined by their wavelength, which is the distance between two consecutive peaks of the wave.

Wavelength

Electromagnetic Radiation

The sun emits electromagnetic radiation energy of many different wavelengths. The radiation affects us in varying ways depending on its wavelength, which is measured in nanometres.

A nanometre is a standard international (SI) unit of measurement for electromagnetic radiation.
1 nanometre = 0.000,000,001 metres

CATEGORY	WAVELENGTH IN NANOMETRES (NM)	RELEVANCE TO LIFE ON EARTH
Cosmic rays	0.000001	Dangerous and potentially cancer-producing, but penetrate to Earth only in insignificant amounts
Gamma rays	0.0001	Dangerous and potentially cancer-producing, but penetrate to Earth only in insignificant amounts
X-rays	0.01	Dangerous and potentially cancer-producing, but penetrate to Earth only in insignificant amounts; used artificially in medicine
Ultraviolet radiation	100–400	Causes short- and long-term damage to exposed living matter, particularly causing, in humans, sunburn, photoageing and skin cancer
Visible light	400–800	Allows us to see; enables plants to create food molecules; drives human biorhythms; lifts human mood
Infrared radiation	800–17,000	Warms our bodies
Radiofrequency radiation	100,000,000	Has no known significant effect; used artificially for telecommunications

rhythms. Our mood and sense of well-being may also be affected by visible light; deprivation of sunlight can cause a type of winter depression known as seasonal affective disorder (SAD).

Very small amounts of UV radiation also promote the synthesis of vitamin D in the skin. This vitamin strengthens bones and thereby prevents rickets. However, vitamin D also comes in our diet – for example from fish oils, eggs and dairy products – which provides all that we need in normal circumstances. Overall, it therefore seems that the UV radiation part of the spectrum may not be of any value to us at all, but instead is just responsible for most of the harmful effects associated with sun exposure, such as sunburn, photoageing and skin cancer (see pp.33–52). However, UV radiation is also sometimes used by doctors to treat skin conditions if nothing else is effective, although damage to the normal skin still occurs during this form of therapy (see p.82).

UV RADIATION FROM THE SUN

The UV radiation component of sunlight is small but biologically important, consisting of the wavelengths between 100 and 400 nanometres (nm). These are then further subdivided into three categories:
- UVC: 100–290 nm
- UVB: 290–320 nm
- UVA: 320–400 nm

UVC is completely absorbed by the ozone in the atmosphere and does not penetrate to ground level, so the solar UV radiation that reaches us consists only of UVB (up to about five per cent) and UVA (95 per cent or more). These percentages are, however, approximate

How UV Radiation Behaves

The three types of UV radiation behave in different ways because they are of different wavelengths. They therefore have differing effects on us, and these are summarised below.

UVC (100–290 nm) Completely filtered out by the ozone layer and does not reach the Earth's surface

UVB (290–320 nm) Makes up about five per cent of the total solar UV radiation around midday in summer, but is responsible for 80–90 per cent of sunburn, photoageing and skin cancer

UVA (320–400 nm) Makes up about 95 per cent of the total solar UV radiation in summer, but accounts for just 10–20 per cent of UV-related skin damage. However, it plays an important role in the development of abnormal skin reactions to the sun, the most common of which is polymorphic light eruption (prickly heat)

overall values and the relative amounts vary considerably with the time of day and year, latitude and other factors (see p.16).

Although UVB accounts for only a small proportion of the total solar UV radiation, it is nevertheless extremely important because these UVB wavelengths are the ones that are mainly responsible for causing sunburn, photoageing and cancer of the skin. This is because they are many times more effective than UVA in causing harmful changes to the genetic material of living cells, namely DNA (see p.29). As a result, even though UVA comprises most of the total solar UV radiation throughout the year, it is generally responsible for only about 10–20 per cent of the harmful effects of sun exposure. There is clear evidence, however, that regularly exposing your skin to high-dose UVA from sunbeds causes damage similar to that resulting from exposure to sunlight, although sunbeds often emit a great deal of UVB as well. UVA also plays an important role in the development of a whole host of abnormal skin rashes caused by the sun (see pp.72–85).

OTHER SOURCES OF UV

Although the sun is by far the most important source of UV radiation on Earth, UV is also emitted artificially by many fluorescent and other lamps, and also by arc welding equipment, and these may be an important source of exposure for people who work with them. Special UV radiation lamps are also designed for careful use under medical supervision on skin conditions such as psoriasis and eczema. Many people are also further exposed in their workplace or at home to very low intensity UV radiation from fluorescent lights. As a result of the minimal UV output involved, however, these types of lights are not generally believed to cause measurable skin damage. On the other hand, tungsten halogen spot lamps are potentially dangerous if used continually, as they can cause sunburn after minutes to an hour or so of exposure, and they probably also have the potential to cause photoageing and perhaps skin cancer after many years of constant use.

HOW UV LEVELS VARY

The factor that has the greatest influence on the intensity of terrestrial UV radiation is the height of the sun in the sky, which depends on the time of day, the season and the latitude. Altitude, cloud cover, terrain

Variation in UV Levels Throughout the Day

UV radiation levels vary with the distance the sun's rays travel through the atmosphere. Peak levels occur when the sun is most directly overhead.

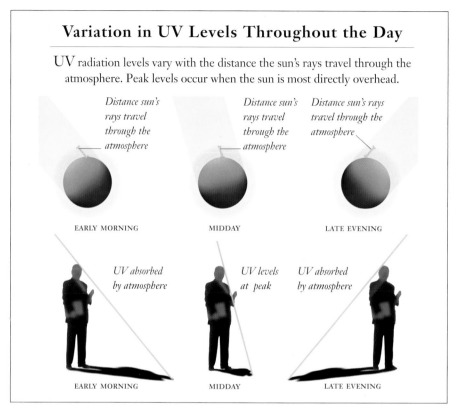

Distance sun's rays travel through the atmosphere

Distance sun's rays travel through the atmosphere

Distance sun's rays travel through the atmosphere

EARLY MORNING   MIDDAY   LATE EVENING

UV absorbed by atmosphere

UV levels at peak

UV absorbed by atmosphere

EARLY MORNING   MIDDAY   LATE EVENING

and the amount of sky that is visible are modifying factors of less importance.

TIME OF DAY

The highest levels of UV radiation are received within the four hours encompassing the solar zenith (that is when the sun is at its highest point in the sky). In the UK, this is between 11:00 and 15:00 on a cloudless day in summer. At this time, the angle of the sun relative to the Earth's surface is such that sunlight has the shortest distance to travel through the atmosphere and the least opportunity to be absorbed or deflected. As a result, about one-third of the total daily UV radiation is received between 12:00 and 14:00 and three-quarters between 10:00 and 16:00.

The levels of UVB in particular vary significantly during the day, being much more susceptible to the atmosphere's effects than those of UVA and visible light; thus, the UVB intensity increases and then decreases by many times between 10:00 and 16:00 in summer. In practical terms, therefore, this means that the risk of sunburn is greatest when the sun is at its highest, usually around 13:00 in the UK, Europe and USA, although you still need to keep skin exposure to a minimum between around 11.00 and 15.00 in summer, as radiation levels are persistently high during this period.

An easy rule of thumb is that if your shadow is shorter than your height, you should not be exposed to the sun unprotected. Early in the morning and later in the day, however, when shadows are longer, there is much less harm from sunlight.

SEASON

Seasonal variations in UV radiation intensity, particularly of UVB, are most pronounced in temperate climates such as in northern Europe, including in the UK. In these regions, UVB intensity can vary by up to 25-fold between winter and summer. The strength of UVA, however, is more constant, being less susceptible to reflection, deflection and consequent weakening during a longer or shorter passage through the atmosphere. On the other hand, nearer the equator levels vary much less, being high all the year round because the sun is

Seasonal Variations in UV Levels

The Earth's axis of rotation is tilted in relation to the plane in which it travels on its annual cycle around the sun. There are therefore seasonal variations in the sun's intensity as one hemisphere and then the other tilts towards the sun.

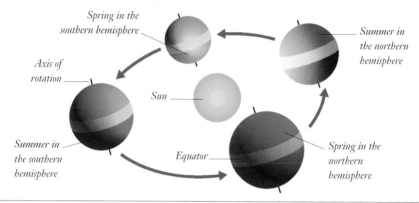

always relatively high in the sky in the middle of the day, regardless of the time of year.

GEOGRAPHICAL LATITUDE

The further you are from the equator, the less UV radiation there is. For example, the average annual exposure of a person living in Hawaii (20°N) is approximately four times that of someone living in northern Europe (50°N). This increase in exposure is again caused by the decreased distance that UV radiation has to travel through the Earth's atmosphere at lower latitudes.

ALTITUDE

As a general rule, for every 300 metres (around 1,000 feet) of increase in altitude, the ability of UV radiation

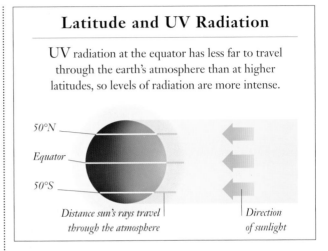

Latitude and UV Radiation

UV radiation at the equator has less far to travel through the earth's atmosphere than at higher latitudes, so levels of radiation are more intense.

50°N

Equator

50°S

Distance sun's rays travel through the atmosphere

Direction of sunlight

to cause sunburn increases by about four per cent. This is because the radiation passes a shorter distance through the atmosphere to reach mountainous or other high-altitude areas.

CLOUD COVER

Clouds usually reduce the amount of UV radiation reaching the ground only moderately, having a proportionately much smaller effect than they do on temperature, so you can still burn easily on a cloudy summer's day, even if it feels cool. This is because the water in clouds absorbs heat much better than it absorbs UV radiation. For this reason, scattered clouds in a blue sky make only a small difference to the levels of UVB, although complete light cloud cover can, on occasion, reduce the likelihood of sunburn by up to about 50 per cent, and very heavy clouds can reduce it by as much as 90 per cent. In other words, it is usually possible to burn on a summer's day even when the weather is cloudy, cool and dull. Pollution has a similar effect to clouds, again reducing the effects of UV radiation just a little.

WIND

Wind, unless very warm, has the falsely reassuring effect of reducing your skin temperature so that you feel cool even though UVB levels are unchanged. You can therefore get as badly sunburned in a breeze as you can without one. The risk is especially high on a cloudy day when the sun is dull. This is because you are more likely to be unaware of the strength of the sun and therefore may stay out longer.

WINDOW GLASS

Most glass used for windows and car windscreens blocks UVB but not UVA or, of course, visible light. This means that, although such glass markedly reduces the risk of sunburn, it does not prevent UVA-induced skin rashes and long-term damage.

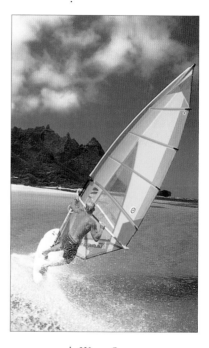

WATER SPORTS
Rippling water and rough seas reflect UVB when the sun is high, so sailing or windsurfing increases the risk of sunburn.

SURFACE REFLECTION

Some surfaces reflect UV radiation well, allowing more of it to reach your skin and increasing your risk of sunburn. Thus, grass reflects only about three per cent of UVB, whereas a dry, white, sandy beach reflects up to about 25 per cent. However, although calm open water reflects no UVB when the sun is high, rippling water and rough seas may reflect much more, perhaps up to 20 per cent. This means that you can get sunburned much more quickly on a beach, even under a parasol, or when sailing, than in your back garden. This sunburn risk may then be increased still further by radiation scattering from the sky (see opposite).

Fresh snow also reflects large amounts of UVB, up to 85 per cent, which, together with the altitude and misleading cooling effects of wind and weather, accounts for the often severe sunburn experienced by unwary skiers.

Risk Factors

Several factors influence the intensity of sunlight and its potential to cause sunburn, photoageing and skin cancer:

- Time of year: the risk is greatest during the summer months, when the sun rises higher in the sky.
- Time of day: the risk is greatest between the hours of 11:00 and 15:00 in the UK, when the sun is highest in the sky.
- Geographical latitude: the risk is greatest near the equator, where the sun always rises high in the sky.
- Cloud cover: the risk is greatest on a cloudless day. Although light cloud only mildly reduces this risk; even heavy cloud removes only 50–90 per cent of the radiation.
- Reflection: the risk is greatest near reflecting surfaces, including sand, snow and rippling water.
- Wind and water: the risk of skin damage is not affected by the cooling effect of either of these.
- Amount of sky visible: the risk is greatest when a large amount of sky can be seen; up to two-thirds of UVB radiation arrives indirectly at all angles from the atmosphere (scattering) rather than just direct from the sun, so the risk may be reduced by as little as a third if the sun is directly obscured but wide expanses of sky are still visible.

TEMPERATURE

The ambient air temperature (for example, 0°C versus 30°C), or the temperature of any water in which you may be swimming, unless you are on a dive at least several feet below the surface of the water, has little influence on the intensity of any incident UVB radiation.

SCATTERING FROM THE SKY

UV radiation does not pass smoothly through the Earth's atmosphere but undergoes many collisions with air molecules on the way, much as snooker balls may behave. As a result the rays reach the ground at all angles from the sky; visible light and heat are affected much less by this process. Therefore, you are still at risk of burning and other skin damage from UVB if you can see lots of sky, even if you are well protected from direct sunlight by clouds, trees, buildings or a parasol. In fact, up to two-thirds of UVB arrives in this way, and only about a third to a half comes in a direct line from the sun.

OZONE AND SKIN CANCER

Ozone is a gas in the upper atmosphere created from oxygen by solar UVC radiation; the ozone then absorbs some of the UVB, which turns it back to oxygen again. At present, therefore, there is a balance between the production and destruction of ozone; the absorption of all UVC and some UVB in the process prevents much noxious radiation from reaching the Earth. If, on the other hand, this currently absorbed radiation did reach us, vast numbers of vulnerable single-celled organisms that are part of food chains, such as plankton in the oceans, would very probably die and possibly end all life.

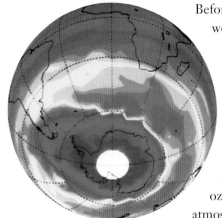

The Ozone Hole
This false-colour image shows total ozone levels. Red and yellow indicate high ozone concentrations, while blue indicates low levels. The white circle indicates an ozone 'hole' over Antarctica.

Before this disaster happened, however, we would all face increased risks of sunburn, photoageing and skin cancer, although we could significantly minimise these by taking more care outside.

It is now well known that certain chemicals and gases, predominantly synthetic chlorine and fluorine compounds used as aerosol propellants and coolants in fridges, are able to alter the ozone balance if they are released into the atmosphere, where they inactivate the ozone. In 1974, when scientists first saw that this was in fact beginning to happen, they also realised the resultant potential for an increase in UV radiation intensity at the Earth's surface. Now ozone 'holes', areas of relative depletion, have repeatedly been recorded by scientists from the British Antarctic Survey during the South Polar spring; the problem is more severe in this region because of the extreme cold, which intensifies the process of inactivation. For the moment, however, ozone loss elsewhere in the world and at other times of year, when UV radiation intensity is high enough to matter, is much less. Nevertheless, there is considerable concern that the phenomenon will become much more widespread unless measures are taken to reduce the pollution responsible on a worldwide scale. Fortunately, however, major steps in this direction are indeed now being taken.

In summary, therefore, despite annual periods of ozone depletion in some parts of the world, particularly over the Southern Hemisphere, there has not been a great deal of evidence of corresponding significant increases in terrestrial UVB levels over the past decades.

If the antipollution measures referred to previously do indeed continue to be adopted, no real increases are now likely to develop; if they are ignored, however, the risk of future major problems remains extremely high.

It is therefore clear that other factors have more to do with the rise in human skin cancer over the last 50 years than any increased UVB levels as a result of ozone depletion. Probably the most important of these is that we now spend much more of our increasing leisure time in the sun, while the increasing age of the population and improved diagnostic techniques are also likely to be significant.

KEY POINTS

- The intensity of UV radiation depends largely on the time of day, the season and the latitude.
- The ozone layer of the atmosphere, which filters out the solar UV radiation most harmful to living matter, is now being slowly depleted by man-made chemicals.
- Terrestrial levels of UVB have not significantly increased.
- The increasing incidence of sun-induced skin damage is probably largely due to recent lifestyle changes.

How UV radiation affects your skin

The skin is the largest organ of the body, weighing about four kilograms and covering about two square metres. It helps maintain body temperature, prevents dehydration and protects us well (if not completely) from harmful environmental agents, particularly infectious organisms (bacteria and viruses, or 'germs'), dirt, dust and sunlight.

THE SKIN
The skin, which is the largest organ of the body, helps to maintain body temperature, prevents dehydration and protects us from the environment.

The skin is also, of course, extremely important in terms of our appearance and in enabling us to receive sensory input from around us. Finally, it helps to dispose of any organisms that do penetrate and probably also helps to destroy early skin cancers.

The skin is made up of several layers, each of which has a specific function:

● The stratum corneum: this is the outermost protective layer – a horny strip of inert dead cells created from the underlying epidermis; these are continuously rubbed off to be replaced from below.

● The epidermis: this 'brick wall' of living cells known as keratinocytes gradually moves up and matures to form the stratum corneum.

● The dermis: this lies beneath the epidermis and acts

The Structure of the Skin

The skin is a complex organ consisting of several layers, each of which has a specific function. Specialised cells, called melanocytes, in the base of the epidermis, produce melanin, a UV-absorbing pigment that gives us a tan.

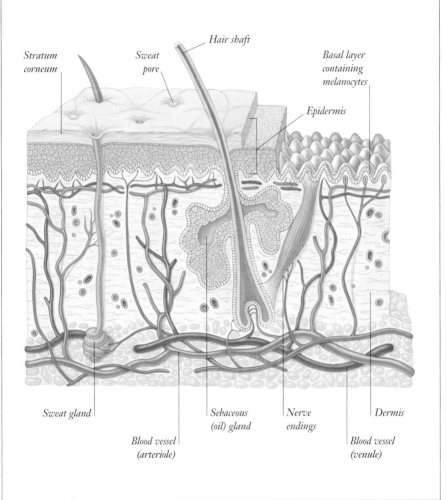

Stratum corneum

Sweat pore

Hair shaft

Basal layer containing melanocytes

Epidermis

Sweat gland

Blood vessel (arteriole)

Sebaceous (oil) gland

Nerve endings

Dermis

Blood vessel (venule)

as a supportive and supply layer, carrying sensory and other nerves and blood vessels to supply the skin with nutrients and oxygen.

- The hypodermis: this lies below the dermis and essentially acts as a protective buffer joining the skin to the body itself; it contains connective tissue and fat.

In more detail, the superficial stratum corneum is tough and inert, helps prevent dehydration and protects the underlying living epidermis from mild to moderate injury, including UV radiation damage and penetration by 'germs'.

The epidermis beneath contains several cell types, particularly keratinocytes, which form the building blocks of this layer and change as they move upwards to form the stratum corneum. At the base of the epidermis are evenly scattered melanocytes, which produce melanin, a UV radiation-absorbing pigment; this gives us a tan. A third type of cell are the cells of Langerhans, which are an important part of the skin's defence or immune system against infection and tumours. Like most cells, keratinocytes, melanocytes and the cells of Langerhans have a central nucleus that contains their genetic programming material or DNA. Damage to the DNA, particularly in those cells that continuously bud off new cells eventually to form the stratum corneum, is thought be important in the development of skin ageing and cancer. Such damage is generally caused in the skin by UV radiation, but it may be augmented by exposure to various chemicals, particularly cigarette smoke.

The dermis lies under the epidermis and consists of a network of supportive fibres, blood and lymphatic vessels, hair follicles, nerve endings and sweat glands.

Collagen and elastin provide fibrous networks that give strength to this layer, and provide the skin with overall elasticity, shape and firmness.

Beneath the dermis is the hypodermis, containing loose connective tissue and fat. This essentially binds the skin to the rest of the body, while also providing a degree of protection against damage from above.

UV RADIATION AND THE SKIN

Approximately five per cent of the UV radiation hitting the skin is reflected, the remainder passing into the tissue, being scattered and then passing out again, or else being absorbed by molecules in the various layers of the stratum corneum, epidermis and dermis. The short-wavelength UVB (290–320 nm) is largely removed in the stratum corneum and in the epidermis, particularly by DNA and melanin, whereas the longer UVA wavelengths (320–400 nm) are mostly transmitted to the dermis to be absorbed there predominantly by haemoglobin in the blood, or else reflected back up and out of the body.

UV radiation has many effects on skin as a result of its absorption by a variety of skin molecules, called chromophores, the most important of which is DNA. After UV absorption, this essential structure undergoes a variety of possible chemical changes, the best recognised of which results in the formation of what are known as pyrimidine dimers. If these are not then rapidly repaired, they are highly disruptive to cells, stopping them from functioning normally and hindering cell division. Further, it is now known that even minute amounts of sunlight on the skin, less than that required to cause sunburn, can often cause DNA

Cell Damage Caused by Sunlight

UVB radiation from the sun can damage DNA, the genetic material in cell nuclei. Most cells repair themselves but release chemicals that can contribute to skin ageing; a few cells mutate and replicate to lead to skin ageing or cancer; a few cells die.

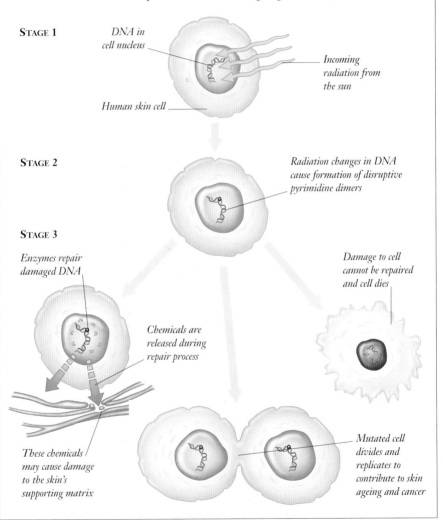

STAGE 1

DNA in cell nucleus

Incoming radiation from the sun

Human skin cell

STAGE 2

Radiation changes in DNA cause formation of disruptive pyrimidine dimers

STAGE 3

Enzymes repair damaged DNA

Damage to cell cannot be repaired and cell dies

Chemicals are released during repair process

These chemicals may cause damage to the skin's supporting matrix

Mutated cell divides and replicates to contribute to skin ageing and cancer

damage throughout the entire thickness of the epidermis. Fortunately, however, most of this damage is repaired within hours to days, although a very small legacy of permanent damage generally remains to contribute to photoageing and sometimes skin cancer.

VISIBLE SKIN DAMAGE

The absorption of UV radiation by skin chromophores (predominantly of UVB by DNA), and the unrepaired damage to the chromophores, are the main cause of later visible skin damage, particularly sunburn, photoageing and skin cancer. Such damage is in fact initiated at all levels in the skin, but, because the UVB is largely absorbed high up before it reaches the dermis, most of the immediate damage that we eventually perceive is to the epidermis, although both UVB and UVA do cause deeper damage as well.

When DNA is damaged by UVB, one of three things happens. The most likely is that the cell accurately repairs the damage through a sophisticated and complex series of specialised enzymes. At the same time, chemicals are also released that are important in the repair of damage to other skin molecular structures and which, as part of that process, cause the underlying blood vessels to swell. These events are what we perceive as sunburn, one example of the general tissue repair process of inflammation (see p.33). The chemicals may also perhaps contribute to damage to the collagen and elastin fibres in the dermis, thus helping to accentuate skin ageing, although direct radiation damage to these fibres and nearby DNA probably plays a part as well (see p.28).

The second possibility, and one that of itself rarely has any serious consequences for the person concerned, is that the damage is so extensive that the cell cannot repair itself and dies. This happens particularly after severe sunburn, for example when your skin blisters and peels.

Finally, the most serious situation is that the damaged DNA is inaccurately repaired. This results in the insertion of a new and very possibly error-producing piece of DNA into the cell, which is passed on when the cell divides. Such an alteration is called a mutation, and it is the step-wise accumulation of these, mostly in the basal layer of the epidermis, that may eventually lead to skin cancer in susceptible people (see p.47). In addition, this mutation process, in less severe form, also contributes to skin photoageing, as mentioned previously.

KEY POINTS

- UV radiation readily penetrates the skin and damages molecules, especially DNA in the cell nuclei, which is important for cell function.
- This DNA damage is largely repaired, but some persistent abnormalities remain.
- These abnormalities may then gradually accumulate, leading slowly to skin photoageing or even eventually to skin cancer.

Sunburn, tanning and photoageing

The absorption of UV radiation by skin chromophores (see p.29), and the consequent damage, leads to the cascade of events known as sunburn, through which the body is largely able to repair the defect.

It is thought that the DNA damage itself provides the trigger for this process, inducing the release of special chemicals that bring about the typical pain, warmth, redness and swelling that we all normally experience some hours after too much sun. The visible aspects are, however, largely the result of blood vessel swelling. In fact, sunburn can vary from mild tingling and pinkness to severe blistering and loss of skin; in the latter case, you may also feel generally unwell.

UVB is far more effective than UVA at causing DNA damage, mostly in the epidermis, and it is therefore much more likely to set off the sunburn response. Further-more, the greater the radiation exposure, the worse the sunburn, but just how much damage is done depends on your skin type. Thus, people with darker skins take

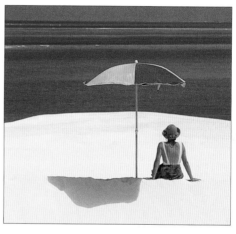

THE DAMAGING SUN
Too much exposure to the sun, for example as a result of sunbathing on a beach, initially causes skin damage in the form of sunburn.

longer to burn than those who are fair (see box opposite), although everybody is susceptible to some extent.

SKIN TANNING AND THICKENING

Exposure to UV radiation also causes the skin to respond in two particular ways. Both of these responses, which are produced as a result of damage to the DNA, have evolved to reduce the sensitivity of the skin to further exposure to UV radiation and minimise further damage.

SKIN TANNING

What we see as a suntan is the presence of brown UV radiation-absorbing melanin pigment in the epidermis. This is released into the epidermal keratinocytes by melanocyte cells of the epidermal basal layer within a few hours of damage to their DNA by sunlight. The pigment is partly transferred to the surrounding basal keratinocytes, clumping protectively above their important cell nuclei, and partly to the keratinocytes above, which then gradually move to the skin surface in the normal way and are eventually shed. This tanning process provides some two to four times greater protection against subsequent UV exposure. This lasts until the tan fades as the superficial skin cells are discarded. Nevertheless, the fact is that a sunlight-induced tan is always associated with UV radiation-induced DNA damage and is maintained only as long as such damage continues to occur. Clearly, therefore, there is no such thing as a completely safe tan other than a fake one or the one that you were born with. Thus, genetically black skin provides around 10–15 times better protection against the sun than white, and brown skin about five times as much.

Skin Thickening

Your skin also becomes thicker within days of sun exposure, and this so-called hyperplasia may last for weeks to months. Again this reaction appears to be a response to DNA injury, this time injury to the basal layer keratinocytes by UV radiation. Thus, within a day or two, once DNA repair has taken place, these keratinocytes begin to divide and multiply much more rapidly than normal, resulting in a several-fold thickening of the epidermis, particularly of the protective stratum corneum, while the dermis also thickens a little. These extra layers can then provide 5–10 times extra protection against the future effects of the sun, especially for the vulnerable basal epidermal layer. This thickening is usually more effective than any accompanying tan, especially in fair-skinned people. The combination of tanning and thickening together however may give up to around 10–40 times increased protection, much better than a tan alone, albeit always at the expense of some permanent skin damage.

── Who Is at Risk? ──

Fair-skinned individuals, especially those with freckles and red hair, burn particularly easily in the sun because of their relative genetic lack of melanin. In fact they sometimes may not tan at all, whereas darker-skinned people will do so with relative ease. How well a tan

The Six Skin Types

Skin types range from those that tend to burn easily and tan poorly to those that are relatively trouble free and rarely burn.

Skin Type	Characteristics
I	Always burns, never tans
II	Usually burns, sometimes tans
III	Rarely burns, always tans
IV	Olive skin, rarely burns
V	Brown skin, very rarely burns
VI	Black skin, virtually never burns

35

develops is thus built into you from birth and depends on which of six arbitrarily defined skin types you have (see box on p.35). People with types I, II or III tend to burn easily and tan relatively poorly, being at greatest risk from the adverse long-term effects of sunlight – namely photoageing and skin cancer, whereas those with types IV, V or VI are relatively trouble-free, except for a tendency to photoageing. Your skin type can thus be readily determined from the way it responds to its initial significant exposure to midday summer sun each year.

PHOTOAGEING

There appear to be two major ways in which skin may age. The first is genetically programmed, so-called intrinsic or normal ageing, affecting the skin all over your body. The second is what is known as photoageing and results from the long-term adverse effects of sun exposure. The degree to which skin photoages is also determined genetically to some extent, in that fair-skinned people who burn easily tend to photoage most rapidly. However, it also depends on how much your skin is exposed to sunlight over the years, whether through normal outdoor activities or sunbathing, or both.

It is possible to judge the effects of any photoageing of your skin by comparing the appearance of the skin on your hips or buttocks with that of your face. Those areas normally covered by clothing are smooth and freckle- and wrinkle-free. Facial

PHOTOAGEING
Long-term exposure to the sun causes the skin to become dry, thickened and wrinkled.

skin, in contrast, may be relatively freckled in susceptible people, namely those with fairer skin, particularly if they have had a lot of previous sun exposure, and, especially in older people, is often dry, thickened, yellowish, blotched brown, deeply wrinkled and covered with thread veins. Allowing for the normal effects of ageing, the difference between skin that is usually covered and skin that is normally exposed is the result of photoageing.

WHAT CAUSES PHOTOAGEING?

Photoageing is the result of accumulated skin damage caused by UV radiation over many years. Just as for sunburn, it is UVB wavelengths that have the greatest effect. However, UVA exposure can also cause changes, although with a tendency to be deeper. These may affect you if you spend a lot of time on a sunbed or sun-bathing using a sunscreen that blocks mostly UVB.

When the body is unable to fully repair damage to the DNA in the cells of the epidermis and the dermis, their structure deteriorates with changes that seem irre-versible. In addition, the chemicals released during sun-burn appear also to harm the dermis, especially causing damage to the network of collagen and elastic fibres that form the major support for the skin and help to keep it wrinkle-free, although this damage may recover over time. These fibres may also be directly damaged by UV exposure. All this means that your skin tends to become gradually drier, rougher and thicker, and thread veins and wrinkles also slowly develop.

Sunlight also causes changes to the melanocytes, which gradually stop functioning in a consistent fashion so your skin may develop a brown blotchiness; it may gradually yellow as well. Finally, your epidermis may become thinner and more fragile. All these changes together are the visible signs of skin photoageing.

Other factors besides sunlight exposure may also contribute significantly to skin ageing, and these include most particularly cigarette smoking.

CAN PHOTOAGEING BE PREVENTED?

In theory, photoageing can be prevented. If you could protect your face from the sun all the time, it should remain relatively young-looking and wrinkle-free into old age. In the past, however, this has not tended to happen, particularly because people have not understood the cause of photoageing.

First, therefore, it is vital to begin any protection programme very early in life: it has been estimated that up to 50 per cent of our total UV radiation exposure is acquired by the time we reach 18 and 75 per cent by 30. We can therefore very much improve the outlook for our children's skin by acting now. As far as adults are concerned, although the time-clock for photoageing has already been ticking for some time, we can very definitely minimise further changes by being careful in the sun from now on (see p.53).

Second, it seems likely that skin photoageing steadily develops even with recurrent minor UV exposure. Thus, increasing evidence suggests that even walking to and from the office or shops, or hanging out the washing, may expose our skin to enough sunlight to cause some photoageing; the skin does not need to burn, or even turn pink, for slow permanent damage to take place.

PROTECT YOUR SKIN
A wide-brimmed sun hat can help to reduce the process of photoageing by shielding your face from direct sunlight.

This therefore means that preventing photoageing probably requires even more effort with regard to sun protection than does preventing sunburn.

In summary, therefore, any steps that you take now to cut down the time you spend outside unprotected will reduce the speed and extent of your eventual photo-ageing, whenever you may start. Although the skin on your face may not look as young as that on your buttocks, it can still look much better than if you do nothing at all to protect it. Also, the younger you are when you start your protection programme, the better your outlook. Further, since you also need to reduce the time your skin is exposed even to ordinary daylight each day, rather than simply making sure you do not get sunburned, you might consider using certain types of make-up and moisturisers now available that incorporate sunscreen ingredients, particularly if you normally use such products or are happy to start. For more information on the prevention and treatment of sun damage and photoageing, see p.62.

KEY POINTS

- Sunburn is a skin repair process.
- Tanning is the release of UV-protective pigment following UV-induced DNA damage.
- This damage also causes the skin to thicken.
- Accumulated skin damage over many years produces photoageing, in which the skin becomes dry, blotchy and deeply wrinkled.

What is skin cancer?

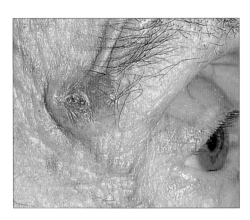

All cancers appear to be made up of body cells that have been gradually damaged through sequential injury to their DNA. This damage makes the cells grow independently of the rest of the body and later infiltrate other tissues.

BASAL CELL CARCINOMA
This form of skin cancer is the most common type. It occurs most frequently on the head and face – parts of the body that receive the most exposure to the sun.

In growing independently, these cells therefore bypass the usual mechanisms designed to prevent this happening. They are dangerous because not only can they damage and affect the normal structures around them, but also they can often later spread through the bloodstream and lymph vessels to disrupt other parts of the body, continuing to grow in these new sites, which are often vital organs such as the lungs, liver and brain. In the long term, they also tend to divert the nourishment necessary for the body's normal activity in order to meet their own requirements.

DNA-damaging agents are known as carcinogens and include chemicals present, for instance, in tobacco smoke, the constituents of certain foods, emissions from radioactive substances, certain viruses and, especially as far as skin cancers are concerned, UVB and UVA in solar radiation.

There are three main types of skin cancer (or carcinoma):
- Basal cell cancers (which are sometimes known as rodent ulcers).
- Squamous cell cancers.
- Malignant melanoma.

The first two types – basal cell cancers and squamous cell cancers – are together known as non-melanoma skin cancers or carcinomas.

The Three Main Types of Skin Cancer

- Basal cell carcinoma
- Squamous cell carcinoma
- Malignant melanoma

In addition, there are two main precursor lesions, solar (or actinic) keratoses, which may precede squamous cell cancers, and lentigo maligna lesions, which may predate one form of melanoma, the lentigo maligna melanoma. Basal cell cancers and other melanomas do not have precursors.

Skin cancers are one of the most common cancers worldwide. In the UK alone there are approximately 40,000 new cases each year; of these, about 28,000 are basal cell cancers, 7,000 squamous cell ones and about 4,000 malignant melanomas. About 2,000 people die each year from such cancers, around 1,500 of them from melanomas. However, most skin cancers are avoidable and all are generally curable if caught early, which is why dermatologists and health campaigners are currently working extremely hard to increase public awareness of all forms of the condition and its prevention (see p.51).

Despite these efforts, there has still been a very substantial increase in all types of skin cancer over the last few decades, with rates doubling approximately every 10–12 years. As stated earlier, this may to some extent be the result of improved diagnostic and disease-reporting techniques, but it probably has more to do with

Deaths from Melanoma

The incidence of melanoma appears related to the severity of solar radiation exposure, and the rising number of deaths suggests people are increasing such exposure.

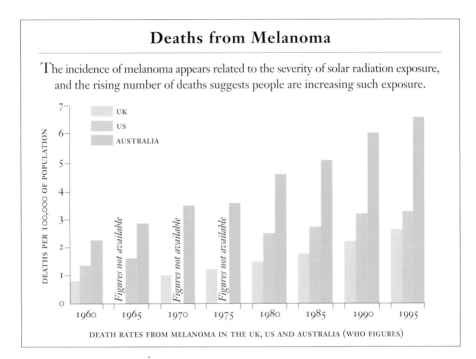

DEATH RATES FROM MELANOMA IN THE UK, US AND AUSTRALIA (WHO FIGURES)

lifestyle changes in recent years. Thus, we now take far more sunshine holidays than we once did, and we may also spend much of our leisure time sunbathing in this country. The possible impact of ozone depletion has not yet been felt, but if unchecked this also has the potential to increase skin cancer risk considerably in the future, unless the apparently effective careful measures referred to earlier continue to be reliably implemented (see p.23). On the other hand, the possible good news is that the annual increases in skin cancer rates appear at last to be slowing, perhaps as a result of the current major efforts at public education.

BASAL CELL CANCERS

Basal cell carcinoma is the most common and least aggressive form of skin cancer, developing from the basal layer of the epidermis. Lesions normally grow slowly, often appearing first as small, flesh-coloured, firm, somewhat pearly nodules, often on the face, neck, shoulders or backs of elderly people. They then slowly enlarge until a central area of broken skin tends to develop; some people first notice the problem when they scratch the lesion, which may then bleed a little and fail to heal properly. Sunlight clearly plays a part in causing this type of cancer, but other factors are also important because not all exposed areas are regularly affected, the backs of the hands particularly being spared. In addition, although people over the age of 50 most commonly develop the disorder, it can also occur in much younger people. The main danger from basal cell cancer is its potential to erode the skin and underlying tissues very gradually over a number of years, although fortunately it almost never spreads to the rest of the body. The treatment is straight-forward if undertaken early and is explained on p.64.

BASAL CELL CARCINOMA
This basal cell carcinoma on the nose of an elderly man appeared over a two-month period.

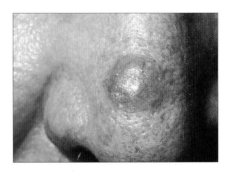

SOLAR KERATOSES

Solar (or actinic) keratoses result from the early disordered growth of groups of keratinocytes in the epidermis. They generally appear on skin, particularly fair skin, that has been continually exposed to the sun over long periods, such as the face, ears, backs of the hands and scalps of men with thinning hair.

Solar keratoses are very common – as many as a third or more of fair-skinned people over the age of 60 have them, particularly those in sunnier climates. They are usually less than a centimetre across, reddish or brownish, scaly or rough, slightly uncomfortable if knocked and sometimes easier to feel than to see. You can check by running your fingers or the palm of your hand lightly over your skin – they feel slightly rough compared with normal skin. There are of course many other causes for rough skin, but any persistent patches on exposed areas just might be solar keratoses.

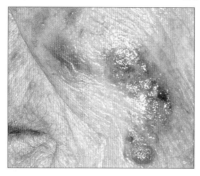

SOLAR KERATOSIS
Solar keratoses are very common, especially in areas of the world that receive high levels of sunshine. Although it is rare for them to do so, they can develop into squamous cell carcinoma.

Solar keratoses are potential precursors of squamous cell carcinoma, but in practice they only rarely progress in this way; thus only 1–2 percent ever become malignant and some may actually disappear, particularly if sun exposure is later minimised. Failing that, however, their treatment is relatively straightforward, by either freezing them or cutting them out, and is detailed on p.63. It is generally worthwhile to have such treatment so as to avoid the slight risk of future squamous cell cancer, as well as to get rid of the often unsightly, slightly sore patches.

SQUAMOUS CELL CANCERS

Squamous cell carcinoma is the second most common type of skin cancer and also develops within the keratinocytes of the epidermis. This disorder is rare in people under 50, and it most commonly affects relatively fair-skinned individuals who have been exposed to regular sunlight over long periods of their lives, perhaps because they have lived in a very sunny climate or else worked or had a hobby outdoors for many years. Typical lesions are slightly tender, reddish or brownish, slowly growing, persistent lumps on any regularly exposed skin; generally they are more bulky and rougher to the touch than basal cell cancers, unless ulcerated. They generally start off as very small patches, sometimes in the form of solar keratoses. You should always consult your doctor about any lump or sore of this type that starts in this way and fails to heal over weeks to months. The treatment of squamous cell cancers is straightforward and described elsewhere (see p.65). Except in the latest stages, treatment generally leads to a complete cure.

SQUAMOUS CELL CARCINOMA
This is the second most common type of skin cancer. It most commonly occurs in fair-skinned people who have been exposed regularly to the sun over many years.

MALIGNANT MELANOMAS

Malignant melanoma is the rarest skin cancer, making up about 10 per cent of the total, but it is also the most dangerous, causing around 75 per cent of all deaths from skin cancer. If caught early, however, as with all other skin cancers, it is readily curable, so it is extremely important to look out for and recognise the early signs of this aggressive condition. It in fact consists of a collection of cancerous melanocytes, the pigment-producing cells of the basal epidermis, and generally appears as a mole larger than about six millimetres across (the size of the blunt end of a pencil), which then irregularly enlarges and darkens over several months; consult your doctor promptly if you have any lesion that behaves like this. Many melanomas seem to develop within pre-existing moles, while others

45

appear to arise in previously normal skin. The condition is much more likely to affect those who are very fair, who tend to freckle easily, who already have lots of moles and who have been sunburned frequently. Younger age groups mostly get them on the trunk (in men) and on the lower legs (in women), whereas very elderly people may also develop them on the face in a relatively less aggressive form; this often follows months or even years of the presence of an initially harmless, fixed, irregular and brown

ABCDE Guide to Melanomas

The ABCDE guide summarises the signs to look out for if you are to identify a melanoma. These changes often occur together and continue to progress over a period of months.

A=ALTERATION IN APPEARANCE OF A MOLE. Ordinary moles do not change. You should therefore consult your doctor if one has permanently altered, particularly if it is continuing to do so; it may have grown darker, bigger or more irregular in outline, or commonly all three.

B=BORDER IRREGULARITY. Ordinary moles generally have well-defined, relatively smooth outlines, whereas melanomas often have irregular or ill-defined edges. Repeated BLEEDING or itching of a mole over more than a week or so, in addition to the other features mentioned here, is a further cause for concern.

C=COLOUR. Ordinary moles are usually evenly, brownly pigmented with a smooth surface. A suspicious mole, however, often has more than one shade of brown with an uneven surface texture as well. Thus, it may be light and dark brown in different parts, or rarely even have red, black or white areas instead or as well. The precise colour outlines also tend to change over weeks to months.

D=DIAMETER. Many ordinary moles are smaller than the blunt end of a pencil. However, melanomas are generally at least as large as this, that is, more than about six millimetres in diameter.

E=ENLARGEMENT. Ordinary moles do not usually grow over a period of weeks or months, whereas melanomas do.

discoloration called a lentigo, later a lentigo maligna, as mentioned on p.41.

You can develop malignant melanoma at any time, although it is more common in those over 50 and extremely uncommon before the age of 16. However, it is still rare overall, affecting only about one in 15,000 people per year in the UK or around 4,000 in total, although rather more of course among those at greater risk.

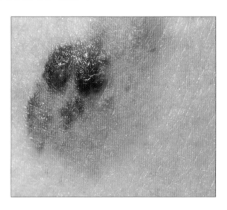

The so-called ABCDE guide (see opposite) summarises the signs to look out for; these changes often, though not always, occur all together and continue to progress over weeks to months.

MALIGNANT MELANOMA
This is the rarest form of skin cancer. It is the most dangerous, however, causing 75 per cent of all deaths from skin cancer.

In addition, many people may develop new, harmless, evenly coloured, regularly outlined, smallish moles from time to time, particularly around the teenage years, but sometimes much later in life as well. These are generally nothing to worry about, but if you have any doubts at all it is best to consult your doctor, particularly as treatment for melanoma is very straightforward in the early stages and almost always fully curative; the procedure is explained on p.65.

WHAT CAUSES SKIN CANCER?

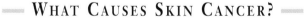

There is now little doubt that the most important cause of skin cancer is excessive exposure of the skin to UV radiation from sunlight, particularly in fair-skinned people. As with sunburn and photoageing, it seems certain that the UVB component of such radiation is the most important contributor. As stated earlier, these

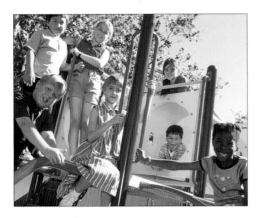

PLAYING IN THE SUN
Although in older life people may often be careful in the sun, the 'time clock' for skin cancer may well have started ticking in their childhood when they may have spent a lot of time outside.

rays are well known to damage skin cell DNA, which governs the structure, growth, function and reproduction of such cells. Therefore, if this damage is severe enough and not repaired accurately, it can sometimes eventually lead to skin cancer, probably through a sequence of changes occurring over a number of years (see p.29). In addition, UVB exposure may also reduce the ability of the immune system to inhibit the development of early cancers, so that any that are triggered during repeated sun exposure may not be eliminated.

As skin cancer is thought to be a step-wise process, probably therefore requiring at least several DNA changes to take place before it develops, there is often a long time lag between any obvious initial damage, such as getting sunburned, perhaps in childhood, and the eventual appearance of any cancer. During this period, more sun damage probably takes place. This time total lag may be up to 30–50 years, particularly for squamous cell cancers, although it may be less at around 10–15 years for basal cell cancers and melanomas. This rate of tumour development is clearly also probably dependent on the amount of continuous sun exposure throughout the days and years, and on the individual's skin type.

Nevertheless, some people who have skin cancer say they never sunbathe or even go out in the sun at all. This seems to be the case particularly in very fair-skinned individuals and is probably because they are very sensitive and repeated sun exposure in their early lives and young adulthood have been the major factors in their cancer development. Other people who work or spend a great deal of leisure time outside may simply pay no attention to whether they are in the sun or not. Thus, just as for skin photoageing, the time clock for skin cancer may be ticking from very early life. Someone who has skin cancer today, for example, may have had a lot of sun while on National Service when young in the Far East, or during a childhood spent on a farm or perhaps through sunbathing every summer as a teenager or young adult. This is clearly not to say that older people need not worry about sun protection – continuing exposure also appears very important in causing the damage that eventually leads to skin cancer. Cutting down on sun exposure at any age is therefore likely to reduce significantly the number of future solar keratoses or skin cancers that may develop.

The relationship between sunlight exposure and skin cancer is most clear-cut for solar keratoses and squamous cell cancers, almost all of which develop on skin that is constantly exposed, such as the face and backs of the hands. For malignant melanoma, however, such a relationship, although still convincing, is less easy to understand. This type of cancer is more common in fair-skinned people with a large number of moles, particularly unusual ones, and in those who have sunbathed intermittently and burned a lot. In addition, melanomas mostly appear on parts of the body that have also been only intermittently in the sun, such as the trunk and lower leg. This suggests that repeated bursts of intense sun exposure that lead to actual sunburn on a number of occasions are likely

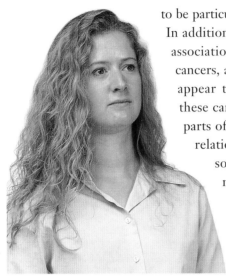

FAIR SKIN
*People with fair skin are
most at risk of photoageing
and skin cancer.*

to be particularly important in causing melanomas. In addition, we do not fully understand the exact association between sun exposure and basal cell cancers, and other factors besides sunlight again appear to be involved (we do not know why these cancers appear more commonly on some parts of the skin than on others); however, the relationship with sun exposure is thought by some to be similar perhaps to that for melanoma.

The very strong association between sun exposure and the development of skin cancer suggests that up to 90 per cent of such cancers could be prevented if people at risk took proper steps to protect their skins carefully from sunlight from an early age (see pp.53–60).

WHO IS AT RISK?

People with skin types I, II and III (see p.35), namely all those with fair skins, are most likely to develop photoageing and skin cancer; the more sensitive the skin, the greater the risk. Furthermore, people who sunbathe, work outdoors for large parts of their life, enjoy outdoor hobbies, such as cycling, gardening, tennis, cricket or golf, or live in sunny climates, especially at low latitudes, are particularly likely to be affected.

As stated earlier, some people with skin cancer may claim never to have sunbathed or worked outside, and therefore wonder how they developed the condition. In most cases, the answer is that they are very fair-skinned and have either been exposed a lot as a child or else have been exposed repeatedly for short periods over many years, usually through routine activities such as walking to and from the office, sitting outside for a sandwich at lunchtime in the summer or gardening. In addition, although not proved conclusively, cigarette smoking may also increase skin cancer risk.

People at risk of melanoma usually also have fair skin, although other factors are likely to be important as far as they are concerned. Thus those with large numbers of moles, particularly oddly shaped ones, and those with a family history of melanoma are especially liable to develop the condition if they have sunbathed and burned a lot. Similarly, basal cell cancers appear to be associated with other, as yet unknown, causative factors besides sunlight, and occasionally with a family history of the condition, although fair skin and frequent sun exposure are again likely to be most important. If you are concerned or in doubt about any of this, you should arrange to see your family doctor or a dermatologist.

── PREVENTION OF SKIN CANCER ──

Skin cancers can largely be prevented. It is estimated that over 90 per cent of such cancers are avoidable by reducing your exposure to UV radiation. You can best achieve this by doing the following, in this order of priority:

• Try to undertake outdoor activities in summer, in tropical climates or at altitude outside the hours of 11:00 and 15:00, namely when the sun is lower in the sky, even on cloudy or cool days. This is even more important if there is a lot of sky visible, or if there is snow, other white surfaces or areas of rippling water nearby. If you must sunbathe, do it outside these hours, when the UV intensity is weaker even if the weather is hot and sunny, and wear a highly protective sunscreen.

● Wear suitably protective clothing where possible, especially a broad-brimmed hat, a longish-sleeved, loosely fitting, close-weave top and similar covering for the legs; in the UK and some other countries, UV-protective clothing is also available, and this may be used instead for greater reliability where desired.

● Routinely use a highly protective sunscreen on exposed skin when outside, particularly between the hours of 11:00 and 15:00 in summer, in the tropics and at altitude. Reapply sunscreen every hour or so, particularly after swimming or exercise.

This advice is even more important for young children who have more sensitive skins, are unaware of the implications of excessive sunlight exposure and have lots of time available to be outside as well.

KEY POINTS

● Continuing UV radiation-induced skin damage, particularly to cellular DNA, leads gradually to skin cancer.

● Fair-skinned people are more likely to develop skin cancer, and especially melanoma.

● Minimising your exposure to UV radiation reduces your risk of developing skin cancer.

Protecting your skin

As we have seen in an earlier chapter, if you are to reduce the chances of suffering from sun-induced skin disorders you need to be particularly careful when the sun is at its most intense (see Solar radiation, pp.11–25).

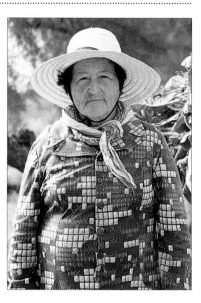

There is a range of precautions that you can take to reduce the exposure of your skin to the sun's harmful radiation, including the following.

TAKE CARE IN THE SUN

The sensible approach is to adopt a Mediterranean or Mexican lifestyle, tending to stay inside around the middle of the day and seeking the shade if outside at such times, as well as covering up with suitable clothes and using a highly protective sunscreen; you may, however, enjoy the outdoors relatively harmlessly at other times.

If you are reluctant to take such precautions because you think they stop you from enjoying the sun, you need to realise that, if you do not, you will almost certainly gradually develop the signs of photoageing – a dry, itchy, blotchy, coarse and wrinkled skin. What is more, you are also putting yourself at increased risk of potentially lethal skin cancer; and both this and photoageing are more

PROTECTION FROM THE SUN
In Mediterranean countries, local people often protect themselves from the harmful rays of the sun by wearing loose clothing and wide-brimmed hats.

likely if you are fair-skinned. All white skins (although not black or, to a lesser extent, brown) are in fact poorly designed to cope with strong UV exposure, and it is most sensible to enjoy being outdoors when the sun is lowish in the sky. Even if it is bright and hot, the damaging UVB will be less intense at these times; although UVA will still be around, this is many times less efficient at causing skin damage. So, cover up with suitable clothes and routinely use a sunscreen during the middle of a summer day, even if there is a cool breeze or a cloudy sky, but be more relaxed for the rest of the time.

Do not forget either that most people in the UK who have indoor jobs get almost half their total sun exposure each year during a single two-week holiday abroad, so you definitely need to be sensible then. However, this does not mean that you cannot enjoy your sunshine holiday as much as before – you just need to take a little extra care!

PROTECTIVE CLOTHING

Until the 1950s, it was relatively common to see people wearing hats – and relatively uncommon to see them sunbathing on a beach. However, changes in fashion and behaviour over the last few decades have meant that we are now increasingly exposing ourselves to the summer sun and are consequently placing ourselves at greatly increased risk of its harmful effects.

If you are out in the midday sun, particularly if you have a thinning head of hair, consider wearing a hat, preferably with a broad brim; this will protect both your scalp and your face from much of the sun's harmful radiation. Also try to wear close-weave, loose-fitting cotton or similar clothing to protect your shoulders, back and arms, and something of similar quality to protect your legs. If you are swimming, windsurfing or sailing, aim to wear at least a T-shirt, which will at least provide some sun protection. Unfortunately, however, such shirts are rather less effective when wet than when dry. Perhaps a better choice in such situations is therefore to wear clothing made from specially designed beach-wear fabrics with a high sun protection factor (SPF) number stamped on them; these are now available in many department stores for children and young adults, providing the same UV protection whether wet or dry.

SUNSCREENS

Sunscreens are skin creams, lotions, mousses and sprays designed to diminish the risk of sunburn by reducing the amount of UV radiation reaching your skin; they also appear to significantly reduce the risk of photoageing and skin cancer if used properly. Sunblock is also a term used in this regard but just refers to more powerful sunscreens – sunblocks tend to be white creams containing zinc and titanium oxide that act a bit like a sheet of baking foil and reflect the sunlight; in spite of the name, however, they still let some UV radiation through! However, all the high protection products are relatively effective if you apply them carefully before sun exposure, reapply them every hour or so, and do not think that using them means you can stay in the sun indefinitely.

TYPES OF SUNSCREEN

There are essentially three types of sunscreen: those containing organic chemical substances that absorb UV radiation, those containing fine inert powders that largely reflect it, and combinations of the two. In the UK, most are combinations and provide protection against

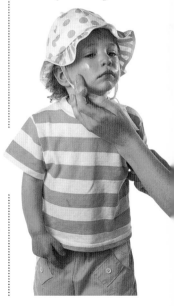

FULL PROTECTION
Children love to play in the sun, and a sunhat, loose clothing and sunscreen are essential if you are to minimise their risk of skin damage.

both UVB and UVA, although relatively less against the latter. However, in other countries this dual effect may not always be present, so check carefully on the packaging. It is now generally agreed that double protection is preferable, although UVB efficacy is certainly the most important.

LEVELS OF PROTECTION

The SPF (sun protection factor) number on the packaging of sunscreens indicates the level of protection against sunburn from UVB, which is by far the most active, and UVA combined, compared with the sensitivity of unprotected skin; the higher the number, the better the protection, the value in fact indicating approximately the number of times that your skin damage is reduced while wearing the preparation. The degree of UVA protection alone is also sometimes stated but is less important; it may be designated by a star rating (* to ****) – again, the more stars the better the protection provided. However, exact UVA protection is not easy to measure and the star ratings are therefore only a guide.

Unfortunately, in many cases, the more effective a sunscreen, the more visible it is on your skin because the stronger preparations contain reflectant products that are not well absorbed. This means that combining a high SPF with good UVA protection and satisfactory cosmetic qualities can be expensive, so the choice you make for best economy depends on what you need from your product (see p.58); newer formulations, however, are becoming more reasonably priced. In any case, a sunscreen of SPF 15–25 with a good star rating is generally best for normal use and is usually also cosmetically acceptable.

Thus, if you are concerned about avoiding sunburn, photoageing and skin cancer, you will need relatively high levels of protection, say around SPF 15–25 with a high UVA star rating.

In addition, a variety of all-year-round moisturising sunscreen products are now available on the market; these appear worthwhile because the skin changes leading to photoageing and skin cancer accumulate with levels of UV radiation exposure insufficient to cause sunburn. In other words, you do not have to burn to build up the steady skin damage necessary for significant long-term effects.

Other effective protective options range from tinted products, which blend in with your skin colour, to brightly coloured preparations designed to look interesting, to water-resistant and hypoallergenic preparations for those with sensitive skins. Ask your pharmacist's advice about the best type for you.

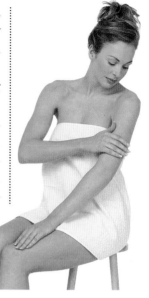

ALL YEAR ROUND
Even if you avoid over-exposure to the sun, you may consider using a moisturising sunscreen daily to protect yourself against the gradual effects of UV radiation.

Sunscreens do have occasional side-effects, but these are generally not serious. They include quite frequent mild irritation soon after application, particularly around the eyes, and rare allergic itchy rashes; if either of these develops, change the sunscreen. Most itchy rashes occurring during sunscreen use are not, however, caused by the product, but represent a form of sun-induced rash (see p.72).

Finally, some people use sunscreens to increase the time that they can stay outdoors uncovered without burning, perhaps to achieve a tan, perhaps just for the fun of it. However, although you may avoid getting burned in this way, you have to accept that such sunscreen use, unless undertaken very carefully, may

Reducing Your Risk of Sun-induced Skin Damage

You can significantly reduce your risk of sun-induced skin damage if you follow these simple guidelines, which need not reduce your enjoyment of being out of doors or on holiday.

- Avoid excessive exposure outdoors around midday in summer or in sunny climates.
- Cover as much of your skin as convenient with suitable clothing when in the sun.
- Wear a cosmetically suitable, combined UVB and UVA sunscreen offering a high SPF (15–25) and high UVA protection (often designated as a star rating – * to ****).
- Reapply the sunscreen every hour or so if you are outdoors for prolonged periods and after swimming, perspiration or exercise.
- Consider also using a sunscreen daily, perhaps incorporated into a moisturiser, on the face and hands, particularly through the summer.

not necessarily provide enough protection to prevent future photoageing or even sometimes skin cancer, especially if you are very fair.

CHOOSING A SUNSCREEN

When you choose a sunscreen, first select products with good sun protection qualities – indicated by the SPF number between 15 and 25 and the four-star (****) rating or another designation of UVA protection – and then decide which product you prefer with respect to other considerations.

If you intend to go swimming, you should check that your sunscreen is water resistant. You might also consider whether it blends with your natural skin colour. Other important considerations might include afford-ability, ease of application, acceptable smell, feel and appearance, and the presence or absence of fragrances or lanolin, as some people are allergic to these substances.

PROTECTION FOR CHILDREN

Children are especially vulnerable to the damaging effects of sunlight for several reasons. First, their skin has had little time to build up the gentle tanning and thickening needed to give a degree of protection (see p.34) and is thus more likely to be damaged. In addition, they do not understand why they should protect their skin by avoiding midday summer sun, wearing hats, covering up and applying sunscreens, so you need to be

What You Can Do to Protect Children

Children are particularly vulnerable to the damaging effects of the sun. There are a number of things that you can do to protect your child from the sun's harmful effects.

- Do not let your baby's skin be exposed to direct sunlight at all and remember that he or she can sometimes burn on sunny days even if he or she is shaded.

- Protect even dark-skinned babies as they too can occasionally burn when young; all young skin needs protection.

- Encourage young children to wear a sunscreen during the summer months, and to apply it carefully themselves. Choose one of the many brands packaged specifically for them with the aim of making it fun. Put appropriate preparations into your child's school bag and enlist the teacher's support where possible to encourage its use before school breaks outdoors.

- Always select products giving high protection (SPF of 15–25 with high UVA protection or star rating) for your children.

- Encourage your children to wear a hat, ideally with some neck protection, during school breaks and whenever they are outside in summer.

- Look at the range of specially designed sun-protective clothes for children; these generally carry a high SPF rating, protect easily exposed parts of the body from direct sunlight (particularly the back and shoulders) and provide the same protection wet or dry.

- Set a good example – behave sensibly in the sun yourself and explain to children why this is necessary.

vigilant on their behalf instead. What is more, they tend to be outside more often than many adults because they have more time to enjoy the outdoors, for example during school lunch breaks.

It is estimated that we receive around 50 per cent of our total lifetime sun exposure by the age of 18 – and it is overall lifetime exposure that leads to skin photoageing and possible skin cancer. It follows therefore that the effort involved in minimising your child's sun exposure while young is very worthwhile, particularly as habits developed early are much more likely to remain than those learnt later. Therefore, by setting an example, and making sure your children understand the dangers of sun exposure, you can lay the foundations for sensible behaviour in the future and help to ensure that they have healthy skin throughout their lives.

KEY POINTS

- You can reduce your risk of skin damage by reducing your exposure to the sun when it is high in the sky.
- Wear loose-fitting clothing and a wide-brimmed hat when the sun is at its strongest.
- Wear a sunscreen to protect your skin.
- Children's skin is relatively sensitive to UV radiation.
- Children are more likely to be exposed to the sun because of their outdoor habits and their lack of understanding of the dangers.
- Take steps to protect children's skin, and teach them to protect themselves for the future.

Treatment

No sun-induced skin damage is particularly easy to treat and it is far better to prevent its development in the first place, if at all possible, by following the advice on protecting your skin given on pp.53–60.

SUNBURN

There is little that can be done to treat the immediate symptoms of sunburn very effectively, and nothing at all to stop any associated long-term damage afterwards; however, if you do overdo things somewhat, the following may help a little until natural healing takes place:

DRINK PLENTY OF FLUIDS
If you are unfortunate enough to become sunburnt, the effects may be reduced at least a little by drinking plenty of non-alcoholic fluids.

• Drink plenty of water and other non-alcoholic fluids, and apply a soothing preparation, such as calamine lotion or aqueous cream, to the affected areas; you can buy both over the counter in pharmacies.

• Take aspirin, paracetamol or any non-steroidal anti-inflammatory tablets, such as ibuprofen, in normal doses as soon as possible after exposure in order to help to ease the soreness until the skin has healed. Ibuprofen gel or similar, although not made specifically for sunburn, may also help a little if applied to the affected skin early enough. Local anaesthetic preparations are also available. Ask the advice of your pharmacist.

• Stay out of the sun for a few days, until the redness and soreness have fully subsided.

• If your sunburn is severe or widespread – for example, if your skin has blistered significantly or you have symptoms such as shivering, headaches or nausea – you should probably consult a doctor or, in particularly severe cases, go to a hospital accident and emergency department. Complications of very marked widespread sunburn can include skin infection and scarring, as well as generalised dehydration, collapse and rarely even death. Over-exposure to the sun can be very dangerous!

PHOTOAGEING

If your skin is already affected by photoageing, you may be able to improve its appearance to some extent by using simple moisturising creams regularly to help relieve the associated dryness and smooth out any wrinkles, but you must remember to use them every day. In addition, there is some evidence that daily use of creams containing vitamin A derivatives (called retinoids), and in particular Retinova® cream containing tretinoin, available on prescription, may slowly reduce irregular pigmentation and smooth out fine wrinkles to a small extent.

Cosmetic or plastic surgery by an appropriate surgeon can also help in a more invasive, expensive and perhaps occasionally risky fashion, in many cases dramatically smoothing out wrinkled, sagging areas of skin. Relatively mild, often effective treatments for brown blotchiness and thread veins include cryotherapy (see p.70) and cold point cautery, respectively, usually

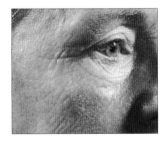

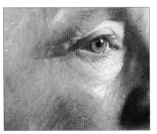

WRINKLE REDUCTION
Creams containing retinoids, substances derived from vitamin A, can help to reduce the wrinkles that result from photoageing if used regularly.

available from a dermatologist. If these are not helpful, other more aggressive treatments for the same problem are chemical peels and laser therapy, the latter also being particularly effective for wrinkles. However, this treatment leaves the treated areas extremely red and raw for days to weeks, and you will also need to take into account the cost and the slight risk of permanent scarring before deciding to go ahead. Discuss it carefully with your dermatologist or surgeon first.

SKIN CANCER

The treatment of skin cancer depends on its precise type and location on the body. Regardless of which treatment you are offered, however, you will always be strongly advised to cut down considerably on future sun exposure. Thus, the fact that you have had skin cancer already means that the sun-exposed skin on other parts of your body is also likely to have been significantly damaged over the years, and you are therefore at high risk of developing another skin cancer if you continue letting too much sunlight get to your skin.

SOLAR KERATOSES

There is a minor degree of debate among doctors as to whether the treatment of solar keratoses offers enough benefit in terms of reducing future skin cancer risk to be worth doing, as so many older people have them and relatively few progress to cancer. However, it does appear that at least 1–2 per cent do advance, especially if the person concerned does not reduce his or her sun exposure from then on, and most people also find the lesions unsightly and itchy or sore. Therefore, it is generally agreed that solar keratoses should be removed once established, and you should consult your doctor if you have any suspicious patches. Treatment usually means the use of cryotherapy (see p.70), a localised freezing spray of compressed nitrogen gas that is generally very effective.

Creams that kill pre-cancer cells are available on prescription and may also be recommended on occasion. These must be applied regularly over several weeks, during which they kill the abnormal but not the normal skin, although they may make the surrounding area annoyingly red and sore for a few weeks. Staying out of the sun thereafter then appears to help to prevent the development of new solar keratoses.

Finally, it is certainly most important to have solar keratoses treated if you are on drugs that tend to suppress your immune system, such as cyclosporin or azathioprine (mostly prescribed after organ transplantations but occasionally for other reasons), because these drugs greatly increase the risk that affected areas will progress to skin cancer.

BASAL CELL CANCERS

Small basal cell cancers can also be treated with cryotherapy (see p.70), but cutting them out surgically or removing them by radiotherapy (see p.70) is much more reliable for larger ones. Sometimes, this type of cancer may slowly come back after any treatment, and a similar, but perhaps slightly more aggressive, approach will often be needed for a final cure. Basal cell cancers do not spread to other parts of the body, however, except in extraordinarily rare instances, and the only real trouble with them is the way they look and their tendency to erode very slowly into nearby structures.

SQUAMOUS CELL CANCERS

Squamous cell cancers are most often treated by surgery, except sometimes in difficult-to-reach skin sites or in very frail people, when radiotherapy may be used instead (see p.70). It is then unusual for the condition to come back, although up to about five per cent do reappear. Very rarely, spread of the cancer may also occur to other parts of the body, such as nearby lymph glands in the neck or armpit, for example, or very occasionally the lungs, bones or brain. Additional surgery and chemotherapy may then discourage further growth. It is generally cancers that have been left for a very long time, and become particularly large locally, that cause problems, although lesions of the lip or ear, or lesions in individuals whose immune system is suppressed by certain illnesses or medications (see opposite), are also likely to spread if not dealt with early. If you have a growth that you think might be a squamous cell cancer, you should see your doctor as soon as possible so that any such problem can be dealt with before the chance of spread.

MELANOMAS

Melanomas are virtually always treated by surgery. They are generally cut out under local anaesthetic and their removal almost always leads to a permanent cure. The usual procedure is that any suspicious lesion is removed first with a narrow margin of normal skin for careful examination under the microscope. If a melanoma is confirmed, a larger area may be taken out at a separate visit to ensure no tumour remains. Occasionally the area will require skin grafting, but more often you will just be left with a larger scar.

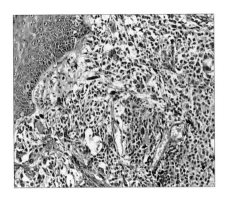

MALIGNANT MELANOMA
Magnified by a microscope, the cells of this tumour appear in a range of sizes, many of them containing large, dark-stained nuclei. Many cells contain the pigment melanin.

If you have a melanoma, you should discuss the matter in some detail with your dermatologist or surgeon. The vast majority of such tumours are, however, thin and non-invasive, do not recur and give no further trouble. Nevertheless, some deeper tumours do have a risk of recurrence or may spread to other areas of the body through the lymph vessels or bloodstream. It is therefore often a good idea to make a further appointment to see your doctor some weeks after your surgery, when you have had time to think, during which period you can make a list of any questions you want to ask. For example, you might now want to be told about your own specific risk of recurrence or spread, whether the event might alter any possible future decision to have children or whether you might conceivably develop another tumour. If necessary, see also 'Useful Addresses' (p.90) for contact details of the Macmillan Nurses, who specialise in the care of people with more persistent melanomas.

After treatment, anyone who has had a melanoma will normally have regular check-ups in the clinic by their dermatologist or surgeon about every six months for five years, or sometimes longer. At these visits, the scar and local lymph nodes will usually be examined for any sign of possible recurrence; usually there is not any. A cancer that does reappear in the same place, however, is often treated with further surgery, which is frequently successful. If, on the other hand, the condition has spread to the local lymph glands, these can usually also be removed effectively by surgery, although chemotherapy may be given at this stage to help prevent further cancer spread.

This is because the drugs used in this technique are able to destroy cancer cells wherever they may be in the body.

Although rare, melanoma is potentially the most aggressively lethal skin cancer; however, early diagnosis and prompt removal are almost always fully curative.

DIAGNOSTIC AND TREATMENT PROCEDURES

The type of skin cancer is first diagnosed following its removal by a skin biopsy. Once the type of cancer has been confirmed by studying the excised lesion under a microscope, any remaining cancer can be treated by further surgery, radiotherapy, photodynamic therapy or cryotherapy. These techniques are described below.

SURGERY – THE SKIN BIOPSY

You will probably need to undergo a special procedure called a skin biopsy to establish the precise diagnosis of your condition. This is a simple technique that removes part or all of a tumour for microscopic examination to determine what cancer it is and, particularly if large, what treatment is best to dispose of it. Usually, however, the abnormality is fully removed during the biopsy, and the tissue is then just examined to check the diagnosis and that all of the cancer has indeed been taken away. If the margins of the lesion are very close to or impinge on the removed skin edges, however, your doctor may well need to excise more tissue to remove the cancer cells completely. If the cancer is large, on the other hand, or awkward to remove completely because of where it is, only a small piece of skin may be taken at first just for microscopic examination; a further procedure will then probably be planned for later.

The Skin Biopsy

A biopsy involves removing part or all of the suspected tumour. The sample of tissue is taken for microscopic examination to aid diagnosis of the form of cancer.

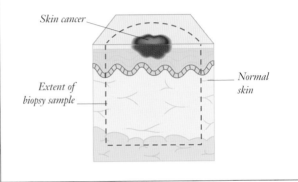

Skin cancer

Extent of biopsy sample

Normal skin

The skin biopsy procedure itself is relatively simple and normally requires no special preparation on your part; you can eat and drink normally beforehand and as soon afterwards as you wish. Furthermore, it usually takes only 10–30 minutes to perform and the local anaesthetic used generally does not cause nausea, drowsiness or other side-effects. As long as you feel comfortable, therefore, there is no real reason not to drive home or go back to work afterwards if you wish. However, many people prefer to take the day off just in case they find the event a strain or any minor soreness afterwards is annoying; they may also arrange for someone to drive them home.

You should inform your doctor beforehand if you are on any medication, particularly steroids, aspirin, non-steroidal anti-inflammatory drugs or warfarin, all of which may conceivably interfere with healing or cause increased bleeding during the procedure. You should also alert your doctor if you have ever had an adverse reaction to an anaesthetic, although this is rare, or if you are allergic to any other relevant substances, such as sticking plaster. Finally, you should mention if you have any heart valve abnormalities or replacements, because you may require antibiotics at the time of the biopsy.

The local anaesthetic used for the procedure is generally a liquid that is gently injected through a fine needle into and around the area to be removed. You can usually briefly feel the sharpness of the needle, some skin areas being more sensitive than others, and often also a little stinging as the anaesthetic goes in, but this rapidly passes and thereafter there should be no discomfort. As the effect wears off an hour or so later, however, you may again experience a little soreness, aching or tenderness at the biopsy site, but this is usually mild and can be eased if necessary by taking paracetamol.

After the event, the removal site will usually be closed with stitches and covered with a dressing. All you then have to remember is to keep the involved skin carefully clean and dry. You will probably also have to go back to your doctor four to 14, or occasionally more, days later to have the stitches removed. However, if the wound oozes or bleeds more than just slightly after the operation, you may need to see your doctor sooner and may perhaps need a pressure pad or further stitch for the wound. If you develop significant pain or swelling at the operation site over the next few days, you should again consult your doctor sooner because the area may have become infected, which then interferes with healing. If this does happen, a course of antibiotics will usually solve the problem, or else occasionally the stitches may need to be removed early.

RADIOTHERAPY

Although most forms of skin cancer can be cured by surgical removal, occasionally this may not be the best approach, particularly if the lesion is large or in a place that makes removal awkward, or if the person concerned is very old or frail. In these circumstances, therefore, radiotherapy may be used instead; this generally involves the use of superficial X-rays over a short course of treatment to destroy the abnormal cells. In addition, some normal tissue is damaged and whiteness, superficial scarring or spider veins may sometimes occur and persist at the treated site, although generally there are no other important side-effects.

PHOTODYNAMIC THERAPY

In rare instances, photodynamic therapy may be used to treat skin cancer; this is still an experimental procedure, however, and your doctor will therefore explain it fully beforehand if it is being considered. The technique involves the use of a photosensitising chemical, a porphyrin precursor, which is usually injected into a vein or applied directly to the affected skin, after which it is taken up just by the cancer cells because they are the most active. When visible light is then applied to the affected area over a course of treatment, it is absorbed by the chemical and destroys the cancer, generally causing a little soreness or burning, but no other problems. However, people who have had treatment may be advised to avoid daylight for several hours afterwards, as the skin may remain very sensitive to burning for that length of time.

CRYOTHERAPY

For most solar keratoses, and some small or superficial basal cell cancers, the preferred treatment is often cryotherapy, sometimes after a biopsy to confirm the diagnosis. The technique is relatively simple and involves freezing the lesion on one or several occasions a few weeks apart with a localised spray of liquid nitrogen. A severe cold injury of around -40°C is inflicted on the cancer or pre-cancer cells and kills them. While the treatment is being given, you will experience a moderate to marked burning feeling, which persists for seconds to minutes, after which the skin will be red for another few minutes to hours, then often blistering or sometimes breaking down over a day or so to form a scab. Thereafter, usually over about a further two weeks, healthy skin forms at the damaged sites; it is usually reddish to begin with but later is totally normal. Occasionally, however, the area may become brownish for some weeks or else very rarely permanently pale, especially if a larger lesion has been treated aggressively.

Cryotherapy is generally convenient and effective, being quick, involving relatively little discomfort and virtually never leaving scars but still killing any cancer or pre-cancer cells. It does not, however, penetrate very deeply, and any lesion that is large, of uncertain diagnosis or suspected of being aggressive must be surgically removed or treated with radiotherapy after a biopsy to ensure success.

KEY POINTS

- Prevention of UV-induced damage is the best approach, as sun damage responds relatively poorly to treatment.
- Skin cancers are usually cured by minor surgery or radiotherapy, but delay can allow the cancer to spread.

Sun-induced rashes

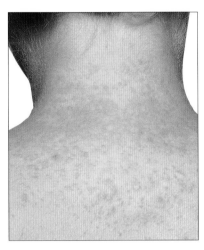

There are some 20–30 forms of sun-induced rash, many of them rare; they are subdivided into groups as described below. Polymorphic light eruption (colloquially called prickly heat) is the most common and is given most attention.

PRICKLY HEAT
In the case of prickly heat, an itchy, red, spotty rash develops within minutes to hours of exposing your skin to spring or summer sun.

ALLERGIC REACTIONS

The most common allergic skin reaction to sunlight is polymorphic light eruption. Other, much rarer allergic conditions are chronic actinic dermatitis, actinic prurigo, hydroa vacciniforme and solar urticaria (see p.75).

POLYMORPHIC LIGHT ERUPTION

About 10–15 per cent of people in the UK have this condition, often incorrectly known as prickly heat because it is caused not by warmth but by UV radiation; about five per cent of Australians, 10 per cent of North Americans and 20 per cent of Scandinavians also have it. More women than men are affected, often from adolescence or early adulthood, although children also develop it occasionally, as well as a few adults in later life. Skin type makes little difference, and black and brown skins are quite frequently affected; there may also be a family history of the condition.

Within minutes to hours of exposing your skin to spring or summer sun, an itchy, red, spotty rash, often like goose-flesh, blisters or hives, develops, often only on some exposed areas but usually symmetrically; it frequently does not affect the face or backs of the hands. The outbreak generally lasts for a few days to weeks before gradually subsiding, provided the skin is protected from sunlight. Most people just have the problem on very sunny days, or once or twice at the start of the sunny season or on holidays abroad, but more severely affected individuals suffer throughout the whole spring and summer.

The exact cause of polymorphic light eruption is not fully understood, but it seems likely that a genetic predisposition leads some individuals to develop a hyper-sensitivity or allergic reaction to a substance in the skin that is chemically altered by UV radiation and thereby appears foreign to the body. In people who do not have the inherited predisposition, the body apparently fails to react to these altered substances.

Many people with polymorphic light eruption never consult their doctor; either they have learnt to live with the condition, or they avoid strong sunlight. For others, however, it can be an extremely distressing condition. Nevertheless, it is generally readily treatable and, if you are bothered by it, one or several of the following measures virtually always work:

● Avoid exposing your skin to sun known by you to be strong enough to induce the condition.

● Cover susceptible skin with suitable clothes when you are outside.

● Use a high SPF sunscreen that provides good UVA protection as well.

If these measures are not enough, see your GP, or if

he or she cannot help, ask to see a dermatologist. At this stage, the diagnosis must be confirmed because other sunlight-induced conditions (such as lupus, see p.80) may produce similar abnormalities; none is, however, quite like polymorphic light eruption. After this, you might have preventive treatment if you wish, which, in 60–90 per cent of cases, stops the rash appearing for several months to a year or two before further treatment may be needed. This treatment comprises a several-week course of twice-weekly, low-dose, UV radiation exposures at the beginning of spring or before a holiday; it is available in many hospitals (see p.82).

Paradoxically, such an approach seems to correct the allergic response but is too low a dose to do any harm, apart from occasionally inducing the rash temporarily after which the treatment may still be effective anyway. The treatment is then repeated, if necessary, annually for at least the next few years, after which permanent tolerance may occasionally set in. If therapy is unavailable, inconvenient, ineffective or unnecessary because of the rarity of your attacks, however, a final, usually very useful treatment is to have a corticosteroid injection or course of tablets, available from your GP or dermatologist, for a few days, as early as possible in an attack. This will usually settle it rapidly. Such treatment may be used up to about every three to four months if required; more frequent or lengthy courses have the potential occasionally to cause a gradual build-up of side-effects. Brief treatment every now and then rarely causes trouble, indigestion and minimal depression being all that might happen; in this case the medication should be stopped and the effects rapidly disappear. For frequent rashes, however, phototherapy is needed instead.

Rarer Allergic Reactions to Sunlight

Treatment for all these conditions includes avoiding sunlight, covering up with appropriate clothing, using a sunscreen and sometimes preventive phototherapy (as described opposite for polymorphic light eruption). If phototherapy is insufficient, oral medication may often be tried.

- **CHRONIC ACTINIC DERMATITIS**: a very infrequent condition usually affecting older men, especially those who have had considerable previous sun exposure and have current outdoor hobbies, such as gardening. It mostly affects the face, neck and backs of the hands with a persistent eczema, caused and readily maintained by UV radiation.

- **ACTINIC PRURIGO**: a rare, persistent, scratched, spotty, sun-induced rash of the arms, legs and face, mostly in children, which worsens in the summer.

- **HYDROA VACCINIFORME**: a very rare, blistering, scarring, sun-induced eruption that usually affects children; otherwise behaves similarly to polymorphic light eruption.

- **SOLAR URTICARIA**: a rare, recurrent, nettle rash-like eruption, usually with the hives running together, which comes on within minutes of sunlight exposure and subsides within an hour or two of covering up.

RARE DNA REPAIR DISORDERS

Another, rare, group of conditions causing sensitivity to the sun are the DNA repair disorders.

XERODERMA PIGMENTOSUM

This is the most common of these disorders. It usually causes a strong tendency to sunburn, often with severe blistering after very little sun exposure, and to very early photoageing and skin cancer. This is because people with this condition cannot effectively repair the skin DNA damage caused by UV exposure as a result of inheriting defective repair genes. If you suspect that your child may have this condition, see your doctor; treatment is difficult but not necessarily impossible.

▪ CHEMICAL AND DRUG SENSITIVITY ▪

Some externally administered chemicals and drugs can increase the sensitivity of the skin to UV radiation. There is also a group of rare conditions – the porphyrias – in which the skin is instead sensitised to sunlight by internally produced chemicals called porphyrins.

THE PORPHYRIAS

The porphyrias are predominantly, but not solely, inherited disorders, the most common being porphyria cutanea tarda. This generally affects people of middle age, causing skin fragility and scattered, occasional blistering of sun-exposed skin, usually on the backs of the hands. This happens because internally produced porphyrins, the chemical building blocks of the red haemoglobin pigment in blood, accumulate and absorb too much UV and visible light in the skin, thereby being stimulated into damaging the surrounding tissue. It is therefore important to consult your doctor if this seems to be happening to you because the condition is usually treatable; if nothing is done, however, liver damage may develop in some instances. Just occasionally, excessive sunbed use may cause a similar condition, but this does not lead to liver damage.

A rarer type of porphyria, which causes a much greater degree of sun sensitivity, is known as erythropoietic protoporphyria (EPP). This generally starts in early childhood and is associated with a very severe, painful, burning skin sensation within minutes of being outside in the summer. Again this happens because excessive porphyrin in the skin absorbs UV and

PORPHYRIA
In porphyria cutanea tarda the skin becomes fragile, and sun-exposed skin, usually on the backs of the hands, can become blistered.

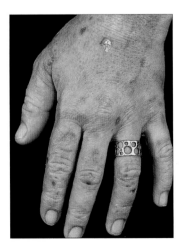

visible radiation, leading to nearby tissue damage. If a child is too young to tell you that his or her skin hurts, the only sign of this condition might be crying whenever the child is in the sun. Any child who reacts in this way should be therefore seen by the family doctor and, if necessary, by a dermatologist in case EPP may be the cause. Treatment is difficult but not always impossible.

REACTIONS TO DRUGS AND CREAMS

There are also a large number of oral medicines and skin preparations that can increase skin sensitivity to UV radiation in a variety of ways. Most often they cause sunburn-like inflammation, or sometimes blistering, of skin that has been exposed to the sun, but there may be other problems, such as a burning sensation without a rash, skin fragility with scattered blisters, eczema or, occasionally, nail abnormalities. Generally, the sensitivity develops within days to weeks of starting a new medication, unless perhaps this is in winter and you do not see much sun for some time; spring is then the time that the trouble usually starts.

Common medications causing such sensitivity are listed in the box on p.78, but there are many others, so if you think your skin is affected as described after starting a new drug you should consult your doctor. Furthermore, pharmaceutical manufacturers give their particular formulations of drugs a trade or brand name, in addition to their approved generic or scientific name. Thus, if you suffer from any of the conditions in the table and are taking a medication for it, you should look for the generic/scientific name of the substance on the packaging or the leaflet inside (usually in small letters), to check if it is indeed on the list.

Drugs and Photosensitivity

Some drugs taken orally to treat common medical conditions can increase the sensitivity of the skin to UV radiation in certain people, most commonly causing sunburn-like inflammation.

MEDICAL CONDITION	PHOTOSENSITISING DRUGS (GENERIC OR SCIENTIFIC NAME)	
High blood pressure (hypertension)	Amiloride Bendrofluazide	Chlorothiazide Frusemide Nifedipine
Depression/anxiety	Amitriptyline Doxepin Imipramine	Chlorpromazine Haloperidol Dothiepin
Pain	Naproxen	Piroxicam
Bacterial infections/acne	Doxycycline Oxytetracycline	Minocycline Sulphamethoxazole Isotretinoin
Diabetes	Chlorpropamide	Tolbutamide
Heart disease	Amiodarone	Captopril Quinidine
Epilepsy	Carbamazepine	
Skin conditions	Preparations containing fragrances, particularly bergamot oil, sandalwood, or lavender	

However, most people can take these medications without developing sun sensitivity, and those who do often experience only a mild reaction.

The treatment of drug photosensitivity is by changing the drug, restricting sunlight exposure, using a sunscreen regularly or perhaps in some cases just taking the medication at night, if that is medically appropriate.

DISORDERS AGGRAVATED BY SUNLIGHT

There are many skin conditions that are not actually caused by sunlight but which may sometimes be aggravated by it, although some are more likely to improve after exposure. Some people with eczema, for example, which is mostly lessened temporarily by sunlight, find the sun makes their skin itch more or otherwise makes the eczema worse, even in cool conditions. However, it is more common for heat (from the sun or a fire, for example) to have this effect rather than UV radiation and, if this happens to you, you may need specialist investigations to determine which sunlight component is actually responsible. Other conditions that may also be aggravated by sun exposure include acne and psoriasis, although again many people who have these conditions find that their skin improves in summer.

No one knows exactly why these conditions are made worse by sunlight in some people, but UV radiation may perhaps alter the skin immune processes causing the diseases, or else sometimes add further sunburn-like inflammation to an already angry and sensitive skin.

The main approach to therapy is to have treatment for the underlying condition, as well as cutting down your exposure to sunlight, and be scrupulous about applying a sunscreen. Sometimes, courses of low-dose preventive phototherapy, as for polymorphic light eruption, may also be helpful, except in people who have lupus (see below), when the condition may instead be made worse.

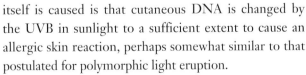

OTHER CONDITIONS

There are several other skin conditions affected by sunlight. These include lupus, vitiligo, albinism and melasma.

LUPUS

This particularly well-known sunlight-aggravated disorder is best recognised for its hallmark, if rather rare, abnormality of a fixed, butterfly-shaped redness of the nose and cheeks, supposedly giving patients' faces a wolf-like look (hence the word lupus, which is Latin

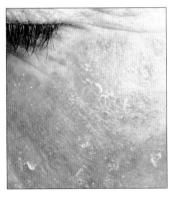

HALLMARK OF LUPUS
This relatively uncommon condition may be associated with redness across the nose and cheeks.

for wolf). Much more common as far as light sensitivity is concerned, however, are flat, scaly, slightly sore red patches, apparently induced by the UVB radiation in sunlight, on other exposed sites. This may be the sum total of the condition, although rarely internal abnormalities such as sore joints and a generalised feeling of being unwell may also occur, again sometimes worsened by sun exposure. The condition is also known to be associated with various immunological abnormalities, and one theory of how the rash itself is caused is that cutaneous DNA is changed by the UVB in sunlight to a sufficient extent to cause an allergic skin reaction, perhaps somewhat similar to that postulated for polymorphic light eruption.

Treatment of the disorder and rash consists of sun avoidance, the use of strong sunscreens and the application of steroid cream. In addition, a variety of oral medications may also be necessary in severe cases, such as certain anti-malarial drugs, steroids, immunosuppressive drugs and even rarely thalidomide. Sometimes the condition may also very gradually settle spontaneously.

VITILIGO AND ALBINISM

Vitiligo and albinism are associated with a lack of the protective pigment melanin in the skin in patches (vitiligo) or all over (albinism) as a result of a predetermined susceptibility. There is thus a marked tendency to easy sunburning of the affected areas. The best advice therefore is to minimise exposure to strong sunlight, cover the affected sites as much as possible with appropriate clothing and use a high factor sunscreen regularly on the exposed skin. Naturally fair-skinned people who have vitiligo will find that protecting the skin as much as possible helps to prevent the normally pigmented sites from tanning and so keeps the contrast between normal and abnormal areas less noticeable.

Albinos need to be especially vigilant, as they can also develop skin cancer relatively easily if careless in the sun, whereas people with vitiligo usually seem not to, for reasons as yet poorly understood. Albinism is present from birth and is unfortunately untreatable. Vitiligo, however, sometimes responds, regrettably often only temporarily, to regular applications of steroid creams or lotions to the affected patches, or else phototherapy, both over a number of months.

MELASMA

Melasma, or chloasma, is a condition that most often affects young and middle-aged women; it is characterised by a patchy brown melanin pigment discoloration, usually of the face, particularly the temples, cheeks and upper lip, but occasionally of other skin. The exact cause is not known, although a genetic tendency and the female hormone oestrogen seem to predispose to the condition. Other factors also apparently involved in triggering it are perfumed substances applied to the affected areas of skin and, most particularly, sun exposure. Some girls first develop the problem around puberty, but the condition is most common after a woman first starts taking the oral contraceptive pill (which contains oestrogen) or during pregnancy, which markedly increases oestrogen levels. The discoloration tends to fade once the pill is stopped or the baby is born; it also helps to minimise sun exposure where possible and to use a sunscreen. Skin preparations containing hydroquinone, prescribable by doctors or available, for example, as FadeOut® over the counter, may gradually decrease the colour as well, if used regularly over several months. Skin irritation, allergy and, in theory after continual use for months or years, an extremely rare orangey discoloration called ochronosis can result from using such products, although FadeOut® is a relatively weak preparation and trouble with it is unlikely. Like all medications, however, it should be used in accordance with the instructions, and if you experience problems you should discontinue its use and seek medical advice.

UV RADIATION THERAPY

As mentioned on p.14, although UV radiation is generally harmful to the skin in the long term, there are a number of eruptions that can be greatly alleviated, albeit usually only temporarily, by its use as a medical treatment. Such conditions may or may not actually be caused by sunlight, and those most likely to respond are psoriasis, eczema, vitiligo and polymorphic light eruption, although a whole host of others may sometimes do so as well. When used in this specific way, the benefits of UV radiation in a particular individual are considered to outweigh the potential risks, even though the treatment does also inevitably involve some overall damage to the skin. The situation is discussed in detail with the patient beforehand, and the treatment, which can only be used for a limited period in total because of the potential build-up of side-effects, is not used without the patient's consent.

There are currently two main types of UV radiation treatment, and these are:

● UVB phototherapy, which is given alone as broad- or narrow-band UVB, which refers in each case to the breadth of the wave-length spectrum emitted by the lamp.

● Psoralen and UVA photo-chemotherapy (PUVA), which is a combination of a photo-sensitising medication called psoralen with broad-band UVA exposure.

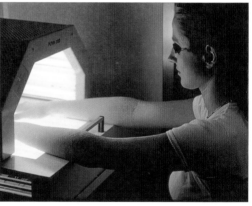

RECEIVING PUVA
PUVA, a combination of a medication called psoralen and UVA phototherapy, may clear certain skin conditions such as psoriasis, albeit usually temporarily.

UVA radiation without psoralen, on the other hand, which is broadly what many, particularly older, sunbeds deliver, is many times less effective at treating skin disease than either UVB or PUVA, and still damaging overall to the skin, and you should not therefore generally use self-therapy with these devices as a substitute for the medically supervised approach.

Before your doctor decides to offer you phototherapy for any skin condition, however, he or she will carefully assess you to make sure that to all intents and purposes it will be safe. You will therefore be asked whether you are on any drugs or medications that might increase your UV sensitivity (see p.77), whether you have had much previous sun exposure and whether you have ever had conditions such as polymorphic light eruption or skin cancer. Your doctor will then explain the advantages and possible risks of the treatment, which include a small chance of burning and a very gradually increasing risk of photoageing and skin cancer if the therapy should need to be continued over a number of years. These risks are, however, now fairly precisely documented and the radiation doses recorded accurately. The twin aims of medical supervision are clearly to keep each treatment dose below that which might cause sunburn and to ensure that your cumulative (or lifetime) exposure is as low as possible overall, so as to minimise the risks of long-term problems.

It is not known for certain how phototherapy improves those conditions responsive to it. However, psoriasis and eczema seem to be disorders in which the immune system is overactive, thereby causing an inflammation leading to the characteristic rash. Phototherapy appears to modify this response, probably by damaging skin immune cell DNA in the first instance, which thereby impedes various subsequent immunological pathways. In addition, it may also slow down normal, although in psoriasis excessive, epidermal basal cell proliferation; in this way, at least in psoriasis, it may help to reduce the skin overgrowth characteristic of the disease; again, it probably does this by its effects on cellular DNA, this time in the basal cells.

In vitiligo, another disorder that is sometimes responsive to phototherapy, UV radiation exposure again probably damps down abnormal immune activity affecting the skin tanning cells (melanocytes) – very possibly a major causative factor in vitiligo – while also stimulating melanin production in those melanocytes still function-ing normally. However, phototherapy is by no means always effective in this condition – many individuals respond slowly or poorly, whereas others relapse steadily and need continuing treatment; the long-term risks of the therapy may then outweigh the benefits. In practice, therefore, it seems that phototherapy for vitiligo is most suited to people with dark skins and relatively few and small affected patches, particularly on the face or trunk.

Finally, the photosensitivity disorder, polymorphic light eruption, probably an immunologically mediated condition as well, also responds, in this case usually very satisfactorily, to short preventive courses of phototherapy, as already described on p.74.

KEY POINTS

- There are many sun-induced skin rashes that affect a significant proportion of people. Polymorphic light eruption (prickly heat) and drug photosensitivity are the most common.

- Polymorphic light eruption responds to several forms of treatment, including low-dose preventive phototherapy.

- UV phototherapy is used under medical supervision to treat a number of skin conditions, but it does slowly damage the skin in the same way as sunlight.

Questions and answers

Do I really need to worry about sun exposure in the UK?

Yes. Between about April and September in the middle of the day UV radiation levels in the UK can be almost as high as those in the Mediterranean; the only real differences are that they do not persist for so long and the brightness and warmth of sun, unimportant as far as skin damage is concerned, may be much less, so making the sun seem less dangerous. This means that you can burn almost as easily during the middle of the day on a British beach as you can on a Spanish one.

If therefore you spend a fair amount of time outside during the summer months in Britain, playing sport or gardening, for example, or if you have a job that means you are outside for much of the year, you can certainly receive enough sun to cause skin cancer, particularly if you are fair, and certainly enough to cause photoageing, without ever going abroad.

What if I want to get a tan?

You cannot sunbathe without causing damage to your skin, however slowly or carefully you build up a tan, so it is better not to aim for this at all. If you have brown or black skin already, you are unlikely to do much harm, but you may not then want to tan! It is a personal choice for you to make, but you should certainly be aware of the risks of sunbathing so that you can make an informed decision.

Sunbathing is at its most dangerous for everyone, but most particularly for fair-skinned people, when the sun is high in the sky, whatever the weather; it is thus relatively safe to sit outside either early or late in the day when the sun is low, even if still warm or bright. Therefore, whether at home or abroad, avoid the sun in the middle of the day where possible, wear suitable clothing to cover you when outside and regularly use a sunscreen of SPF 15–25. You should also realise that a suntan is actually a response to skin cell DNA injury caused by UV radiation. However, this again applies much more to fair-skinned people, and the deeper the tan in such people, the greater the skin damage that has been caused, and thus the higher the risk of photoageing and skin cancer in the future.

It is also important to realise that melanoma, although previously relatively rare, has become increasingly common, and that it is a potentially very serious form of cancer that can be fatal; it is now one of the major causes of death in people in the 26- to 35-year-old age group. There is also a lot of evidence to suggest that it is repeated bouts of sunburn, which are most likely to happen when you are sunbathing on holiday, that are particularly important in causing this type of cancer, particularly again in fair-skinned people.

If you want to have a tan, therefore, there is only one way that you can get it safely and conveniently, and that is to use a fake tanning preparation. These days, as well as being safe, such products can give you a virtually perfect imitation of the real thing. Nevertheless, if you are going to sunbathe anyway, start with short periods of exposure over a few minutes and gradually build up; also use a sunscreen of moderately high protection factor, say 10–15, and stick with that because, if you do burn, it spoils your tan anyway!

Is it safe to use a sunbed?

Sunbeds emit radiation generally very similar to that in midday summer sunlight and therefore have largely the same effects, so you should avoid them altogether. This is because, by using

them, you are really just damaging yourself without even being able to enjoy the outdoors at the same time! However, most dermatologists agree that banning them is as inappropriate as banning cigarettes or alcohol; people should rather be made aware of their potential dangers so they can make an informed choice about using them.

Whether you use older types of sunbed, which emit predominantly UVA radiation, or more modern ones with UVB and UVA together, the effect in terms of skin damage is very similar to that from exposing yourself to the sun. This means that you are risking the same sort of skin damage, which may rarely be in the form of severe or, as has happened very occasionally, even fatal sunburn! There is also a risk of the following problems when you use a sunbed, just as there is when you sunbathe: polymorphic light eruption, lupus, melasma and drug photosensitivity in the short term, and, in the long term, skin ageing and cancer, as well as a form of porphyria-like (see p.76) increased skin fragility. On the other hand, the risk of melanoma from sunbed use has not yet been precisely quantified, but it seems likely that this is also increased, and people with unusual or large numbers of moles should therefore not use a sunbed at all, just as they should not sunbathe. All in all, sunbeds are very similar to sunlight in their potential to cause skin damage and should be avoided. If you do use one, you may get away with it if you are lucky, but you should use it for no more than 20 sessions a year to keep the risk at least moderate.

Is it a good idea to use a sunbed for just two to three weeks a year before holidays to get a bit of a tan and so avoid burning when I get there?

No it is not a good idea to use a sunbed in this way because the damage you do outweighs the value of any tan or protection you might achieve, which is virtually always minimal anyway and equivalent only to a sunscreen of SPF 2–4. Better to use a fake tan and a sunscreen on holiday.

Can sunlight harm my eyes?

Yes, sun exposure is associated with a number of eye problems, including particularly cataracts; for this reason, people having phototherapy for the treatment of skin disease (see p.82) must wear sunglasses. Such cataracts occur with long-term exposure over the years; however, you may also get very sore eyes from severe exposure to bright sunlight, particularly in snow, a condition called snow blindness. Looking directly at the sun for more than a few seconds may also cause permanent loss of sight. Ideally you should wear sunglasses on a summer's day to protect your eyes, while of course also protecting your skin; however, make sure you buy sunglasses that give you good protection against both UVB and UVA.

If I wear prescription spectacles will this magnify the harmful effect of UV radiation on my eyes?

No. Clear glass or plastic normally absorbs virtually all UV radiation, certainly all the UVB, although obviously allowing visible light to penetrate. You therefore need take no major precautions when wearing prescription spectacles unless the light is very bright, in which case for comfort you would do best to wear sunglass attachments or else buy prescription sunglasses.

I know I do not get a suntan from sitting in front of the telly or my PC at work, but am I still at risk from UV radiation?

No, there is no risk from either of these because they do not emit this radiation.

I am of Afro-Caribbean origin and I have a very dark skin; do I need to take any precautions against the sun? Should I be careful with my children in sunlight? Am I at the same risk of photoageing as a fair-skinned person?
You need to take only moderate precautions for yourself at the beginning of summer or a sunny holiday, just to stop early burning, although photoageing certainly does still occur over the years in people with dark skin, and you should thus take care if you wish to avoid that; skin cancer essentially does not occur, however. On the other hand, dark-skinned babies can sometimes burn relatively easily and should therefore be carefully protected until they are older, as described earlier in this book.

I seem to have to put a lot of suncream on my skin to cover it properly. Do these chemicals get absorbed into my body and if so can they do me any harm?
No, careful studies suggest that they do not harm you; however, it is probably wise not to use them excessively in babies up to about the age of six months, by which time their skins have generally become fully mature.

Useful addresses

The British Association of Dermatologists
19 Fitzroy Square
London W1P 5HQ
Tel: (020) 7383 0266
Fax: (020) 7388 5263
email: admin@bad.org.uk
This association represents dermatologists around the country. It also provides members of the public with a list of dermatologists in their area, if required, but does not recommend specific doctors. To consult a dermatologist, it is generally necessary to be referred by a general practitioner.

British Association of Plastic Surgeons (BAPS)
Royal College of Surgeons
35–43 Lincoln's Inn Fields
London WC2A 3PN
Tel: (020) 7831 5161
Fax: (020) 7831 4041
email: secretariat@bats.baps.uk

Cancer Research Campaign
6–10 Cambridge Terrace
Regents Park
London NW1 4JL
Tel: (020) 7317 5027
Fax: (020) 7487 4310
Web site: www.crc.org.uk
Funds research into cancer and education. Provides information to people with cancer and their carers.

Cancerlink
11–21 Northdown Street
London N1 9BN
Freephone: 0800 132905; Freephone (Asian language line): 0800 590415; Freephone (Mac helpline for young people): 0800 591028
Provides information and emotional support for people with cancer and their families. It is also a resource to over 500 cancer support and self-help groups throughout Britain providing training and advice for people setting up support groups.

Eczema Society
163 Eversholt Street
London NW1 1BU
Tel: (020) 7388 4097
Fax: (020) 7388 5882

Health Education Authority
Trevelyan House
30 Great Peter Street
London SW1P 2HW
Tel: (020) 7222 5300
Fax: (020) 7413 8900

Imperial Cancer Research Fund
PO Box 123
Lincoln's Inn Fields
London WC2A 3PX
Tel: (020) 7242 0200
Fax: (020) 7269 3100
Web site: www.icnet.uk
Provides information on cancer
to anyone who requests it.

Macmillan Cancer Relief
Anchor House
15–19 Britten Street
London SW3 3TZ
Tel: (020) 7351 7811
Fax: (020) 7376 8098
Web site: www.macmillan.org.uk
A national charity dedicated to improving
the quality of life for people with cancer
and their families. It funds the Macmillan
Nursing Services for home care, and
hospital and hospice support. Financial
help may also be given.

Marie Curie Cancer Care
28 Belgrave Square
London SW1X 8QG
Tel: (020) 7235 3325
Fax: (020) 7823 2380
Web site: www.mariecurie.org.uk
Runs Marie Curie nursing homes and
provides a community nursing service day
and night. Involved also in research and
the education of health professionals in
the fields of cancer care and prevention.

The Psoriasis Association
7 Milton Street
Northampton NN2 7JG
Tel.: (01604) 711129
Fax: (01604) 792894
Provides information on all aspects of psoriasis, as well as promoting research. It also produces a journal three times a year and organises an annual conference on psoriasis.

Vitiligo Society
125 Kennington Road
London SE11 6SF
Tel: (020) 7840 0855
Fax: (020) 7840 0866
email: all@vitiligosociety.org.uk
Web site: www.vitiligosociety.org.uk
Provides information on all aspects of vitiligo, produces a regular journal and organises meetings and outings for member patients with the condition.

Index

Acknowledgements

PUBLISHER'S ACKNOWLEDGEMENTS

Dorling Kindersley would like to thank the following for their help
and participation in this project:

Design Assistance Chris Walker; **Production** Michelle Thomas;
DTP Jason Little; **Consultancy** Dr. Sue Davidson;
Indexing Indexing Specialists, Hove; **Administration** Christopher Gordon

Illustrations (p.27, p.68) Richard Tibbetts; (p.30) Debbie Maizels

Picture Research Andy Sansom; **Picture Librarian** Charlotte Oster

PICTURE CREDITS

The publisher would like to thank the following for their kind
permission to reproduce their photographs. Every effort has been made
to trace the copyright holders. Dorling Kindersley apologises for any
unintentional omissions and would be pleased, in any such cases,
to add an acknowledgement in future editions.

Colorific p.33; **National Medical Slide Bank** p.76; **Rex Features** p.83;
Salford Royal Hospitals NHS Trust p.62; **Science Photo Library** p.11 (ESA),
p.43, pp.3, 40, 44, 45 & 47 (Dr. P. Marazzi), p.66 (Biophoto Associates), p.80;
Tony Stone Images p.7 (David Harrison), p.21, p.36 (Joe Cornish), p.48 (Charles Thatcher),
p.53 (Richard Passmore); **University of Wales College of Medicine** p.72